Preface

People with intellectual disability (learning disability) can experience a wide range of psychiatric, behavioural, genetic and physical conditions. A psychiatrist working with this group of people needs to have a broad understanding of these conditions, which are often beyond the range encountered when working with the general population. Some disorders occur more frequently in people with intellectual disability, whereas the clinical presentation of other disorders can be modified by the presence of significant intellectual disability itself or be affected by communication problems.

Different conditions frequently coexist, and there is often social and economic disadvantage, all of which have an additive effect on the individual, preventing optimal functioning.

This book examines the concept of intellectual disability, describes the common clinical conditions encountered by the psychiatrist, and concludes by discussing treatment approaches with particular emphasis on teamworking. The purpose of the book is to clarify a complex area of need and to give an overview of the scope and role of the psychiatrist in this field.

The book is aimed at professionals and interested lay people, and it will be of value to doctors in training and other professionals who are seeking to improve their knowledge and awareness of the wide range of problems encountered in day-to-day practice.

Ashok Roy
Meera Roy
David Clarke
September 2005

About the editors

Dr Ashok Roy is a Consultant in the Psychiatry of Learning Disability in Birmingham and North Warwickshire. He is the Medical Director at North Warwickshire Primary Care Trust and a Senior Clinical Lecturer in the Psychiatry Department at Birmingham University. He is the Specialist Health Adviser for the British Institute of Learning Disabilities and is on the Learning Disability Executive of the Royal College of Psychiatrists. His interests include clinical outcome measures, service development, access to primary care services, phenomenology of depression and ethical issues in learning disability.

Dr Meera Roy was involved in the commissioning of comprehensive psychiatric services for a city and sub-regional low-secure forensic services. She has been actively involved in training in the West Midlands region and has been instrumental in increasing training opportunities. She has been active at the Royal College of Psychiatrists and convened the revision of the guidelines for meeting the mental health needs of adults with a mild learning disability. She has published in the area of contraception for women with a learning disability, and has a particular interest in autistic conditions. She now provides a psychiatric service for children with learning disabilities in Birmingham.

Dr David Clark is a Consultant in Learning Disability Psychiatry working for North Warwickshire Primary Care Trust and based at Lea Castle Centre, Kidderminster. His interests include genetic syndromes associated with learning disability, especially Prader–Willi syndrome and Angelman syndrome. He was awarded an MD for his work on behavioural and psychiatric aspects of Prader–Willi syndrome. He is the training programme director for the West Midlands Specialist Registrar training scheme.

The Psychiatry of
Intellectual Disability

Edited by

Ashok Roy
Consultant Psychiatrist
Brooklands, Birmingham

Meera Roy
Consultant Psychiatrist
Greenfields, Birmingham

and

David Clarke
Consultant Psychiatrist
Lea Castle Centre, Kidderminster

Radcliffe Publishing
Oxford • Seattle

Radcliffe Publishing Ltd
18 Marcham Road
Abingdon
Oxon OX14 1AA
United Kingdom

www.radcliffe-oxford.com
Electronic catalogue and worldwide online ordering facility.

British Library Cataloguing in Publication Data

A catalogue record for this book is available from the British Library.

ISBN-10 1 85775 695 9
ISBN-13 978 1 85775 695 1

Typeset by Anne Joshua & Associates, Oxford
Printed and bound by TJ International Ltd, Padstow, Cornwall

Contents

List of contributors

Dr Pru J Allington-Smith MB, DCH, MRCPsych
Consultant Psychiatrist
Brooklands
Birmingham
Tel: 0121 329 4959
Email: Pru.allington-smith@nhs.net

Dr Geraldine M Cassidy MB, BCh, BAO, MRCPsych, MMedSci
Consultant Psychiatrist
The Loft
Bedworth
Tel: 02476 315867
Email: Geraldine.Cassidy@nhs.net

Dr David J Clarke MD, FRCPsych
Consultant Psychiatrist
Lea Castle Centre
Kidderminster
Tel: 01562 859022
Email: Clarkes@sinton.fsnet.co.uk

Professor Sally-Ann Cooper MD, FRCPsych
Professor of Learning Disabilities
University of Glasgow
Department of Psychological Medicine
Gartnavel Royal Hospital
Glasgow
Tel: 0141 211 3701
Email: SACooper@clinmed.gla.ac.uk

Professor Shoumitro Deb MBBS, FRCPsych, MD
Clinical Professor of Neuropsychiatry and Intellectual Disability
University of Birmingham
Department of Psychiatry
Division of Neuroscience
Queen Elizabeth Psychiatric Hospital
Birmingham
Tel: 0121 678 2355
Email: s.deb@bham.ac.uk

Dr Mark Luty
General Practitioner
The Glenkirk Centre
Glasgow

Tel: 0141 944 3716
Email: dr.luty@nhs.net

Dr Verinder P Prasher MRCPsych, MD, PhD
Consultant Psychiatrist
Greenfields
Birmingham
Tel: 0121 255 8009
Email: Vee.prasher@southbirminghampct.nhs.uk

Dr Ashok Roy MA, FRCPsych
Consultant Psychiatrist
Brooklands
Birmingham
Tel: 0121 329 4927
Email: Ashok.roy@nw-pct.nhs.uk

Dr Meera Roy FRCPsych, FRANZCP
Consultant Psychiatrist
Greenfields
Birmingham
Tel: 0121 255 8014
Email: Meera.Roy@southbirminghampct.nhs.uk

Dr Sidhartha Tewari MB, Dip Psych, MRCPsych
Consultant Psychiatrist
Lea Castle Centre
Kidderminster
Tel: 01562 859023
Email: S.Tewari@nhs.net

Acknowledgements

The editors would like to thank Debbie Kenny for processing numerous drafts of the book to short deadlines, and Ameeta Roy for her sketch of the Sally Ann test (in Chapter 4).

Part I

General concepts

This section provides an introduction to the concept of intellectual disability. It provides definitions, classifications and information on prevalence, and it also lists the causes of intellectual disability, an understanding of which aids the development of preventive strategies.

Chapter 1

What is intellectual disability?

David Clarke

Introduction

In the early 1990s the Department of Health adopted the term *learning disability* as the successor to terms such as learning difficulty (which is still used with regard to the education of children), mental handicap, mental subnormality and mental deficiency. The term *intellectual disability* is gaining currency, and is used in the titles of academic journals circulated in the UK and elsewhere in Europe.

The term *disability* is preferable to *handicap*, because it describes the effect of lower than average intelligence in a manner consistent with the World Health Organization (1980) definitions of impairment, disability and handicap. An *impairment* is a loss or abnormality of structure or function, including psychological functioning. A *disability* is a restriction or lack of ability to perform an activity within the range considered normal for a human being. A *handicap* is a disadvantage resulting from an impairment or disability that limits or prevents the fulfilment of a normal role. In other words, a handicap is something which is imposed on a disability which makes it more limiting than it must necessarily be, just as weight or score handicap is added in horse racing or golf. The example of Lesch–Nyhan syndrome can be used to illustrate these concepts further. This is an X-linked genetic disorder (affecting only males), caused by a deficiency of the enzyme hypoxanthine-guanine phosphoribosyl transferase. The enzyme deficiency (the disease) causes altered neuronal functioning (the impairment), resulting in learning disability and neuromuscular problems such as muscular stiffness and movement problems (the disability). The enzyme deficiency also results in a very unusual and severe form of self-injury in which affected individuals bite their fingers and lips, causing severe self-injury. Affected men often try to prevent such injury by self-restraint, as a result of which other people may avoid them in social situations and have low expectations of them (thereby creating a handicap).

The term *learning disability* is also preferred by some users of services. Others dislike most or all of the terms in use. Some service users and caregivers feel that terms such as 'learning difficulty' and 'learning disability' understate their problems, many of which have nothing to do with the ability to learn. One of the reasons for the changes in terminology over the years is that in time these terms acquired pejorative overtones, in a similar way to the term 'spastic' (a term that originally meant increased muscle tone). In the international scientific literature the term *mental retardation* is used. This has been defined as an intellectual impairment, arising in the early developmental period, which may lead to disability (if it significantly affects social functioning) or handicap (if the individual is totally dependent on special services). Mental retardation is the pre-ferred term in North American countries, and has been adopted by the World Health Organization in the Tenth Revision of the *International Classification of Diseases (ICD-10)* (World Health Organization 1992). Here it is defined as a condition of arrested or incomplete development of the mind, which is specific-ally characterised by impairment during the developmental period of skills that contribute to the overall level of intelligence. These include cognitive, language, motor and social abilities.

People with learning disability have an overall pattern of intellectual function-ing at a significantly lower level than that of the general population, with associated impairments in social functioning. The cognitive impairment must have occurred during the period of cognitive development (in practice this is usually taken to mean before the age of 18 years).

Tests such as the Wechsler Adult Intelligence Scale – Revised (WAIS-R) quantify different types of mental ability and group them as verbal and non-verbal scales. Subscales allow effects related to dysfunction of specific brain areas, educational underachievement, etc., to be assessed. The full-scale IQ score resulting from a WAIS-R test has been designed to compare the score of the person tested with the scores obtained from a large population of people of varying abilities. Subscale scores correlate with one another so that a person who scores high on one test tends to score high on the others. However, people with specific learning disabilities and those on the autistic spectrum may show a wide range of abilities. For example, a person with autism may be gifted in mental arithmetic but otherwise functioning in the range of learning disability. Two individuals with the same full-scale IQ may also have different profiles of abilities. The distribution of intelligence is illustrated in Figure 1.1.

Intelligence is normally distributed, like other attributes such as height and weight. This means that, in a typical population, most people will have scores close to average, with few people achieving very high or very low scores (*see* Figure 1.1). IQ tests such as the WAIS-R are therefore constructed and scored so that the average (mean) score is 100 and the standard deviation is 15 points.

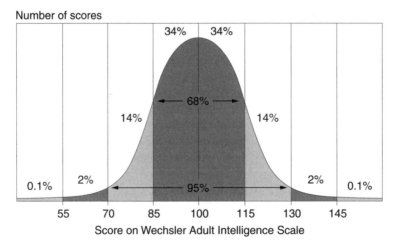

Figure 1.1 Distribution of scores on the Wechsler Adult Intelligence Scale.

Anyone with a score greater than 2 standard deviations below the average (i.e. an IQ of less than 70) can be said to have a statistically significantly low IQ, provided that the test used is appropriate to the person tested and is properly conducted and scored. In some circumstances IQ tests do not provide an accurate assessment of cognitive ability. For example, it would be inappropriate to test a non-English-speaking person with verbal IQ test items in English. Similar considerations apply to other aspects of testing, such as the influence of cultural values and expectations. Despite these potential difficulties, IQ tests are the most accurate method of comprehensively assessing cognitive ability. They are widely used to decide, for example, whether people facing criminal charges should be dealt with through the criminal justice system or within the health service. They are not routinely used to assess cognitive ability in nursing, psychological or psychiatric practice, because less formal methods of assessing abilities and problems are usually more straightforward, less time consuming, less costly and just as effective. Other neuropsychological tests may be needed to obtain information about specific strengths or weaknesses. Assessments of practical skills (such as those carried out by occupational therapists with regard to everyday living skills) may be as important as or more relevant than assessments of global cognitive ability.

The approach adopted by ICD-10 with regard to classification of the severity of learning disability is to describe the typical abilities of people with specific severities of mental retardation (the term used in ICD-10), to allow a comparison with the person who is being assessed. This approach assumes uniformity with regard to the severity of problems (e.g. in self-care skills and language development), whereas some people with learning disability will inevitably have some areas of relative strength and other areas of relative weakness. Table 1.1 summarises the clinical descriptions of different severities of learning disability as outlined in ICD-10, and shows how these relate to the accepted categories of mild, moderate, severe and profound learning disability.

The concept of a mental age is considered by some professionals to be unhelpful. However, as a guide to the kinds of cognitive skills that are usually possessed by people with learning disability the concept has some utility,

Table 1.1 Severity of learning disability and associated problems

Learning disability	IQ	Typical abilities
Mild	50–70	Holds conversation. Full independence regarding self-care. Practical domestic skills. Basic reading/writing.
Moderate	35–50	Limited language. Needs help with self-care. Simple practical work (with supervision). Usually fully mobile.
Severe	20–35	Uses words/gestures to communicate basic needs. Activities need to be supervised. Work only in very structured/sheltered setting. Impairments in movement common.
Profound	< 20	Cannot understand requests. Very limited communication. No self-care skills. Usually incontinent.

provided that its shortcomings are recognised. Adults with mild learning disability are said to have a mental age ranging from about 9 to 12 years. They are likely to have had learning difficulties at school, but many adults will be able to work and maintain good social relationships and contribute to society. Adults with moderate learning disabilities typically have a mental age of 6 to 9 years. They are likely to have shown marked developmental delays in childhood, but can often learn to develop some degree of independence in self-care and acquire adequate communication and academic skills. As adults they will need varying degrees of support to enable them to live and work in the community. Adults with severe learning disabilities have a mental age of between about 3 and 6 years and will probably always need support. Those with profound learning disabilities have a mental age of less than 3 years in adult life. They have severe limitations with regard to self-care, continence, communication and mobility (World Health Organization 1992).

It is important to note that, in clinical practice, a distinction is often simply made between *mild learning disability* (associated with an IQ of between 50 and 69) and *severe learning disability* (with an IQ below 50). In most post-industrial societies people with an IQ of less than 70 are placed at a relative economic (and hence social) disadvantage, and anyone with an IQ below 50 would be most unlikely to be able to live independently or obtain employment. For people with IQs of between 50 and 70, much depends on other factors such as their personality, coping strategies and family support. Some people with mild learning disability do not receive health or social services. The degree to which someone is disadvantaged or 'handicapped' by a learning disability therefore depends on social and cultural factors (and the nature of any associated problems) as well as on the severity of their global cognitive impairment. One of the disadvantages of a label such as 'learning disability' is that it encompasses people with very different problems and needs. Some will have a genetic or chromosomal disorder associated with particular physical (and sometimes behavioural) problems, while others will only have learning problems. Some will have learning problems, but their quality of life will be dependent on factors such as the control of epileptic seizures rather than receipt of services to help with learning problems. However, labels such as 'learning disability' (and diagnoses such as autism or Down syndrome) are helpful in some ways. They provide an 'explanation' of problems, they may reduce feelings of guilt, they may facilitate the provision of appropriate services, and they may serve as an aid to communication between service providers.

How common is learning disability?

The frequency of occurrence of conditions among populations of people is often described in terms of *incidence* (the number of people newly identified as having a condition) or *prevalence* (the number of people identified as having the condition at a particular time or over a defined length of time). For learning disability, the incidence is often described for specific disorders (e.g. Down syndrome) as the proportion of live-born infants who have the condition. The incidence of Down syndrome in the UK is around 1 in 500 live-born infants.

However, such figures may be misleading or may not convey important information. For example, almost all babies with Down syndrome are identified at birth or shortly afterwards. Some other conditions (notably non-specific mild learning disability) will not be detectable at birth, but may become apparent during childhood. Similarly, the incidence of 1 in 500 live births for Down syndrome is an average figure. However, the likelihood of having a baby with Down syndrome rises with increasing maternal age and is about 1 in 32 for women aged 45 years. Only the most severe and obvious conditions, or those for which there is a screening test, are detected at birth. The frequency of learning disability is therefore usually described as a prevalence at a point in time for a defined group of people. Despite the difficulties (e.g. the fact that mildly learning-disabled people may not be identified), there is reasonable agreement from studies in European countries over the past 20 years regarding the prevalence of learning disability. Pooled estimates suggest that about 2% of the population have a mild learning disability and around 0.35% of the population have a severe learning disability. The term 'severe learning disability' is here used to mean all people with IQs that, if measured, would be less than 50.

Associated problems

Problems with learning are often not the most taxing difficulties faced by someone with a 'learning' disability. Conditions commonly associated with learning disability include physical disabilities, sensory impairments, epilepsy (about a third of people with severe learning disability have epilepsy, and the proportion of people with seizures increases with increasing severity of learning disability) and psychiatric disorders. Psychiatric disorders associated with learning disability are considered in more detail in Chapter 3. They include mental illnesses, behaviour disorders, autistic spectrum disorders and behaviours associated with genetic causes of disability.

People with learning disability are also vulnerable to medical problems such as thyroid disorders and gastrointestinal problems. This vulnerability is much more commonly associated with some disorders than with others. For example, people with Down syndrome are particularly vulnerable to thyroid disease and are more likely than members of the general population to develop a dementia of Alzheimer type in middle age. It is important to be aware of the vulnerabilities associated with particular conditions, because treatment may need to be provided, or treatment for another problem modified in order to prevent complications. An example would be the prescription of antibiotics to a man with fragile X syndrome prior to invasive surgical procedures (*see* Chapter 7).

The nature and severity of associated problems often determine the services that will be necessary to allow a person with learning disability to lead as normal a life as possible. A careful balance may have to be struck between risks and benefits. For example, in the treatment of epilepsy, some risk of seizures may be preferable to unsteadiness or cognitive slowing resulting from high doses of anticonvulsant medication. With the advent of newer anticonvulsant drugs, the benefit/risk ratio is improving, but compromises and careful assessments are still necessary.

Multi-axial classification systems

Because learning disability is often associated with physical or behavioural disorders, a system for describing the diagnoses or problems faced by the individual is often more appropriate than a single 'diagnosis'. Such a multi-axial system was developed by the World Health Organization. It has subsequently been modified in the *Diagnostic Criteria for Psychiatric Disorders for Use with Adults with Learning Disabilities/Mental Retardation (DC-LD)* (Royal College of Psychiatrists 2001). The axes used in the DC-LD are shown in Box 1.1.

Box 1.1 Axes in DC-LD

Axis I Severity of learning disability
Axis II Cause(s) of learning disability
Axis III Psychiatric disorders

- **Level A** Developmental disorders (including autistic spectrum disorders)
- **Level B** Psychiatric illnesses
- **Level C** Personality disorders
- **Level D** Problem behaviours
- **Level E** Other disorders

Although designed primarily for use by mental health workers, such a system allows any professional to structure their knowledge about a patient, resident or service user and to communicate this knowledge to others in a succinct format.

References

Royal College of Psychiatrists (2001) *Diagnostic Criteria for Psychiatric Disorders for Use with Adults with Learning Disabilities/Mental Retardation (DC-LD)*. Royal College of Psychiatrists, London.

World Health Organization (1980) *International Classification of Impairments, Disabilities and Handicaps. A manual relating to the consequences of disease*. World Health Organization, Geneva.

World Health Organization (1992) *The ICD-10 Classification of Mental and Behavioural Disorders. Clinical descriptions and diagnostic guidelines*. World Health Organization, Geneva.

Further reading

Fraser W and Kerr M (eds) (2003) *Seminars in the Psychiatry of Learning Disabilities* (2e). Gaskell, London.

Chapter 2

Causes and prevention of intellectual disabilities

Ashok Roy

Introduction

A confusing variety of terms has been used to describe people with what is now called learning disability. Terms such as idiocy and cretinism were replaced by subnormality and handicap. More recently, mental handicap has been superseded by terms such as learning disability and learning difficulty. Some of these terms (i.e. impairment, disability and handicap) have been defined by the World Health Organization (*see* Chapter 1), although they are also used in the Mental Health Act.

Intelligence is normally distributed in the population as shown in the bell-shaped curve in Figure 1.1. This means that the majority of people in the general population have an IQ of around 100 (the arithmetic mean, or average IQ). Smaller numbers of people have lower or higher IQs, and very small numbers have very high or very low IQs. This creates the bell-shaped curve with the highest numbers clustering around an IQ of 100, and smaller numbers at either extreme. The distribution of intelligence is represented in Chapter 1.

Many people with mild learning disability do not have an identifiable cause for their disability. Such people are also much more likely to have parents belonging to socio-economic groups 4 or 5. People with severe learning disability are evenly distributed among the different socio-economic groups at birth, and are very likely to have an identifiable cause for their disability. However, if a person with mild learning disability is born into a family with siblings and parents in socio-economic groups 1 or 2, they are likely to have an identifiable cause for their disability. This illustrates the interaction between genetic influences, which could be regarded as setting a ceiling on possible attainment, and environmental factors, which determine to what extent a person's genetic potential is fulfilled. In practice, the effects of genetic and environmental factors are difficult to separate because they influence and modify each other. Parents from higher socio-economic groups are likely to have more disposable income to devote to books and other educational resources, and may have higher expectations of academic success and different attitudes to schooling and service provision compared with parents from lower socio-economic groups.

Mild and severe learning disabilities are not aetiologically distinct entities. Some studies of people with mild learning disabilities have found that chromosomal aberrations are relatively common, affecting around 19% of cases (Gostason *et al.* 1991). Similarly, not all people with severe learning disabilities have an identifiable cause for their disability (McGuffin 1994).

The causes of learning disability are numerous and complex, and many factors interact to influence the extent of learning disability in adult life. These include factors operating at specific stages of development, including the following:

1   prenatal factors, which affect the development of the fetus before birth and may involve factors that exert an influence before conception, such as exposure of the reproductive organs to radiation
2   perinatal factors, which affect the newborn baby at the time of birth, such as lack of oxygen leading to brain damage and thus learning disability
3   postnatal factors, which affect the child after birth, such as brain damage following measles infection, or lack of stimulation due to the baby's mother being depressed.

Many factors can act at these different stages of development. The nature of the agent, and the time at which it exerts its effect on development, will influence the degree and pattern of learning disability that results from it. Interactions occur so that, for example, infants with causes of learning disability which result in poor muscle tone at the time of birth (e.g. those with Prader–Willi syndrome) are more likely to have complicated births. In such cases the baby may not play a normal role in the birth process and may be vulnerable to additional disabilities resulting from lack of oxygen during birth. Agents may act before, during or after birth to produce learning disability in this way. In about one-third of cases it is not possible to identify the cause of learning disability. It is useful to divide the causes of learning disability into those that primarily affect the child, and those that are secondary to maternal factors.

Prenatal and perinatal factors

Infective or inflammatory agents

The developing fetus can be damaged by a variety of maternal infections. The most common examples are the ToRCH infections (*Toxoplasma*, rubella, cytome-galovirus and herpes simplex). Other infections include those caused by the human immunodeficiency virus (HIV), measles, chickenpox and the bacteria that cause meningococcal meningitis. Sexually transmitted diseases that may damage the developing fetus include syphilis, genital herpes and chlamydia.

Toxins and nutrition

Alcohol consumption and smoking during pregnancy can lead to intellectual impairment. Environmental toxins such as lead have also been implicated, as have drugs prescribed to the mother such as lithium and phenytoin, as well as drugs available over the counter. Diets rich in folic acid can reduce the risk of neural-tube defects such as spina bifida.

Metabolic diseases

These are conditions in which the infant is unable to break down certain substances in the body due to a deficiency of certain enzymes. Examples include phenylketonuria, galactosaemia, maple syrup urine disease, homocystinuria and biotinidase deficiency. There is a build-up of unmetabolised substances which has a detrimental effect on brain development. Research has established dietary folic acid deficiency as a major cause of neural-tube defects such as spina bifida (Department of Health Expert Advisory Group 1992).

Neoplastic processes

Neoplastic processes involve the abnormal growth of tissue, as in the production of cancers or benign tumours. If these processes affect the brain, mental development may be slowed down or show some other abnormality. For example, learning disability, epilepsy and autistic features may coexist in tuberous sclerosis.

Traumatic factors

These include events that occur during the perinatal period or around the time of birth. Mechanical factors such as the use of forceps and hypoxia (lack of oxygen) can result in brain damage. Prematurity, especially when associated with low birth weight, can lead to delayed development.

Chromosomal and genetic disorders

These are of particular importance because they account for an increasing proportion of the causes of severe learning disability, with new genetic techniques being able to detect more subtle abnormalities. The proportion of people with disabilities of 'unknown' origin is slowly declining. The investigation of adults with learning disability must be clinically justifiable (e.g. because appropriate treatment could depend on a diagnosis being confirmed or refuted, or because siblings may require genetic counselling if the learning disability can be shown to be due to a particular condition). These issues are discussed in Chapter 6.

Endocrine disorders

Of all the endocrine disorders, thyroid dysfunction is most commonly associated with learning disabilities. If the under-functioning is picked up at an early stage, thyroxine replacement can usually prevent cognitive impairment.

Autoimmune disorders

Examples include rhesus incompatibility leading to widespread damage to the developing fetus.

Postnatal factors

Infections

Meningitis and encephalitis can cause brain damage, as can infections that lead to dehydration and electrolyte imbalance.

Trauma

Injuries may be accidental (e.g. road traffic accidents) or non-accidental (e.g. violent shaking).

Environmental effects

Inadequate treatment of diseases such as epilepsy, diabetes and hypothyroidism can result in significant brain damage and disability.

Psychological traumas such as neglect and sexual abuse can lead to failure to thrive in infants, or slowed or abnormal development in older children. Social deprivation and lack of stimulation are important influences on development and intelligence.

Maternal causes

These include conditions such as anaemia, hypertension, diabetes and bleeding during pregnancy. They either reduce nutrition to the fetus or lead to premature birth. An unstimulating and deprived environment associated with neglect or abuse has been implicated in developmental delay.

Genetics and learning disability

As discussed earlier, genetic disorders are often responsible for learning disability syndromes. Genetics is the study of heredity and variation in the inherited characteristics of an organism. Genetic material is contained in chromosomes within the nuclei of the cells of an organism. The chromosomes can be seen as thread-like structures within the dividing nucleus, and consist of deoxyribonucleic acid (DNA) combined with proteins. DNA is composed of two chains of nucleotide bases wrapped around each other in a double helix held together by hydrogen bonds between the bases. Each nucleotide has three components, namely a nitrogenous purine base, a pentose sugar and a protein. The four bases in the DNA are adenine (A), guanine (G), cytosine (C) and thymine (T). These can lie in any order along the sugar phosphate backbone. A always pairs with T, and C always pairs with G. Thus one strand contains a sequence of bases that is complimentary to the other, so that each strand can be used as a template to copy the other.

A gene is a length of DNA that codes for the production of a particular protein. Genes are arranged linearly on the chromosomes, each gene occupying a specific position or locus. Other forms of the gene that occupy the same position are called alleles. Each chromosome carries only one allele at a particular locus, although there may be many alleles in the population. In many genes in humans the coding regions (called exons) are interrupted by stretches of non-coding sequences (called introns). Every species has a characteristic number of chromosomes called the karyotype. Humans have 46 chromosomes consisting of 23 pairs, which have the same genetic loci in the same order, although at any locus they may have the same or different alleles. If the same allele is present, the individual is homozygous for the trait, and if the alleles are different the individual is heterozygous for the trait. One member of each pair of chromosomes is inherited from the father and one from the mother. The 22 pairs, which are present in both men and women, are called autosomes. Normally the members of a pair of autosomes are indistinguishable microscopically.

The last pair of chromosomes consists of the sex chromosomes, which differ in men and women. Women have two X chromosomes whereas men have one X chromosome and a smaller Y chromosome. Thus the human male karyotype is described as 46XY and the female karyotype as 46XX. In women each cell contains only one active X chromosome. The other one is usually inactivated and can be seen as a densely staining area called the Barr body in cell smears taken from the inside of the cheek. Chromosome analysis is usually performed on white blood cells which are cultured, spread on slides and stained using different techniques. Banded staining uses dyes that differentially stain parts of the chromosome, producing a characteristic pattern for each pair of chromosomes. Each chromosome has a long (q) arm and a short (p) arm separated by a centromere. Specific chromosomes can be identified by their size and banding patterns.

Mitosis is the process whereby the cells divide, enabling the body to grow and replace dead or injured cells. Meiosis, or reduction division, results in the production of sperm cells and ova. As a result of a mitotic division two cells are formed which are identical to the parent cell, with the full complement of chromosomes, and they are described as diploid. A meiotic division produces gametes (sperms and ova), which contain only one representative of each pair of chromosomes, and are described as haploid. The union of the sperm and ovum restores the number of chromosomes to the diploid state.

Mitosis is a single-stage division, whereas meiosis occurs in two stages. Initially each chromosome divides into two chromatids, and the homologous chromosomes form a quadruple structure. Later both sister chromatids and homologous pairs are separated and pass into four different daughter cells. The disjunction of paired homologous chromosomes is essential for the number of chromosomes to remain constant. Non-disjunction results in abnormalities in the number of chromosomes. Non-disjunction of chromosome 21 leads to trisomy 21 and is responsible for the majority of cases of Down syndrome. Trisomy 18 results in Edward's syndrome and trisomy 13 results in Patau's syndrome.

Aneuploidy is a term used to describe alterations in the number of chromosomes. In Turner's syndrome, affected women have a 45XO karyotype. The karyotype in triple X syndrome may be 47XXX, in Klinefelter's syndrome it is 47XXY and in the XYY syndrome it is 47XYY.

During the meiotic divisions the homologous chromosomes exchange genetic material by breakage and recombination. A whole series of abnormalities can occur during this process. There may be deletions, where a segment of chromosome is lost. Examples of deletions include the cri du chat syndrome, where there is deletion of the short arm of chromosome 5, and Prader–Willi syndrome, where there is deletion in the long arm of chromosome 15. Inversion occurs when a piece of chromosome breaks and is then reattached in the opposite orientation, and duplication occurs when two copies of a segment of a chromosome are produced. Reciprocal translocation occurs when chromosomes of two different pairs exchange segments. In a small number of individuals with Down syndrome the trisomy is due to translocation between chromosomes 21 and 14 or between the two chromosomes of pair 21.

Genomic imprinting refers to the phenomenon whereby the expression of a gene or a set of genes differs according to whether the relevant chromosomes are of maternal or paternal origin. The best-known examples of this are Prader–Willi syndrome and Angelman syndrome, both of which show a deletion of chromosome 15. In the former condition, two-thirds of cases have a deletion on chromosome 15 of paternal origin, while the great majority of cases with Angelman syndrome have a deletion on chromosome 15 of maternal origin. In both syndromes uniparental disomy also occurs, where both members of the chromosome 15 pair are from one parent, so that there is no genetic contribution from the other parent's chromosome 15.

The next important group of genetic disorders associated with learning disability consists of the single gene disorders. The affected genes may be on the autosomes or the sex chromosomes. Several genes may be associated with one disorder, or a single genetic disorder may be associated with several clinical variants. Advances in molecular genetics have helped to localise many of the genes responsible for these conditions.

The inheritance of autosomal disease is dominant when one affected parent passes the condition on to the child. Examples of autosomal dominant disorders associated with learning disability include tuberous sclerosis, Apert's syndrome and mandibulofacial dysostosis. The manifestation of autosomal dominant disease may differ in severity in successive generations.

In autosomal recessive disease the parents are not affected, but both carry the gene and may pass on the condition if their children inherit an abnormal copy from each parent. Important examples of autosomal recessive disease associated with learning disabilities are phenylketonuria, disorders of lipid mechanism such as Tay–Sachs' disease, and mucopolysaccharidoses. In practice, these conditions are relatively uncommon. The frequency of autosomal recessive disease is higher in populations with high rates of consanguinity, such as that resulting from marriages between cousins.

If the genetic abnormality is on the X chromosome, a characteristic pattern of inheritance is seen, with no male-to-male transmission (men always pass on a Y chromosome to their sons). Women may be carriers if they inherit the abnormal X chromosome. They then pass the condition on to their sons. It has long been recognised that men outnumber women with regard to learning disabilities. Fragile X syndrome is an example of an X-linked condition, although its genetics and clinical features are atypical (*see* Chapter 6). Some other X-linked conditions associated with learning disabilities are Lesch–Nyhan syndrome, Duchenne muscular dystrophy and Hunter's syndrome.

A mutation is a change in the base sequence of a gene. It can be either neutral, having little or no effect, or pathological, being associated with significant effects on cellular structure and metabolism. Mutations that occur during the production of sperm and ova cause some of the single gene disorders such as tuberous sclerosis, in which 80% of cases arise as a result of such mutations rather than through inheritance. A number of pathological mutations have been shown to involve variations in the number of trinucleotide repeat sequences, such as cytosine–guanine–guanine (CGG), leading to disruption of gene function. Such unstable DNA trinucleotides have been observed in fragile X syndrome (*see* Chapter 6). Following the mapping of the entire genetic sequence by the Human Genome Project, there has been an increase in the number of conditions for which the genetic abnormality has been identified.

Table 2.1 Primary prevention

Cause	Prevention
Genetic cause	Counselling, screening, amniocentesis
	Termination of pregnancy
Infection *in utero*	Immunisation programmes for rubella, measles
Endocrine and metabolic causes	Screening for phenylketonuria, hypothyroidism, etc.
Nutritional and toxic causes	High-folate diet, avoidance of toxins such as lead and alcohol in pregnancy
Perinatal	Improved obstetric care
Postnatal infections	Early diagnosis and treatment
Accidental injury	Accident prevention
Non-accidental injury	Improved surveillance and early diagnosis
Inadequately treated diseases	Early diagnosis and treatment

A more comprehensive account of genetic factors and lists of psychiatric disorders may be obtained from textbooks of genetics such as *Seminars in Psychiatric Genetics* (McGuffin 1994).

Prevention

Primary prevention aims to avoid the occurrence of a disabling condition. It depends on a knowledge of the causes of learning disability, and the implementation of preventive strategies (*see* Table 2.1).

Genetic and chromosomal disorders

Genetic counselling can provide information on specific genetic conditions, the risk of recurrence and the interventions that are available.

The first step in prevention is the accurate and specific diagnosis of the suspected condition. Once an accurate diagnosis has been made, the parents of the affected child should be given information on the risk of their next child having the condition.

If an adult is affected, similar counselling would need to be given to siblings and other family members. If conception has not taken place, the family needs to have an understanding of the condition that is causing concern, the risk and extent of learning disability associated with it, the mode of inheritance, the carrier status of the parents and the risk of the pregnancy leading to the birth of a child with learning disability.

If conception has taken place, an assessment needs to be made of risk factors such as maternal age, family history and exposure to deleterious environmental factors such as infections in early pregnancy. This may need to be followed by prenatal testing.

- The measurement of maternal alpha-fetoprotein (AFP) is used to detect disorders such as spina bifida, anencephaly and Down syndrome. The test on a maternal blood sample is carried out between weeks 16 and 18 of pregnancy.
- In the UK, women are offered a triple assay of maternal serum alpha-fetoprotein, unconjugated oestriol and human chorionic gonadotrophin at 16–18 weeks of pregnancy. Based on the results, the risk of the fetus having Down syndrome can be calculated and a decision can be made about whether to proceed with amniocentesis.
- Chorionic villus sampling is carried out between weeks 7 and 9 of pregnancy and involves the removal and examination of a part of the placenta for any chromosomal abnormalities.
- Amniocentesis involves the study of cells taken from the fluid surrounding the fetus to detect abnormal chromosomes. This is performed in week 16 on women considered to be at high risk on account of their history or age.
- Ultrasound and fetoscopy are being used to aid detection of congenital malformations.

After a diagnosis has been made, the parents must be helped with sensitivity to make a decision as to whether they want to continue with the pregnancy or terminate it. Some investigations that are associated with a risk to the baby (e.g. amniocentesis) will only be undertaken if the parents are considering termination of a pregnancy in the event of an abnormality being found.

Universal screening of newborn infants for phenylketonuria and hypothyroidism has been effective in reducing intellectual impairment due to this cause. In the USA, by screening healthy adults for Tay–Sachs' disease in populations of Jewish people of Ashkenazi descent, followed by genetic counselling, the condition has almost been eliminated among these populations. It has been suggested that populations at risk of fragile X syndrome would benefit from DNA-based screening (Sabaratnam *et al.* 1994; Slaney *et al.* 1995).

Infections

Widespread immunisation programmes for diseases such as rubella and measles have dramatically reduced the incidence of babies born with handicapping diseases.

Endocrine and metabolic diseases

The prevention of these disorders can be effective if they are detected early and remedial measures are instituted at an early stage. Screening at birth for hypothyroidism and phenylketonuria can lead to replacement therapy or a special diet being commenced immediately, thereby reducing the level of learning disability.

Toxic and nutritional factors

The most effective strategy in the amelioration of these factors is health education and health promotion, with a consequent adoption of healthy lifestyles. Beneficial approaches would include reduction of alcohol intake and cigarette smoking, improvement of maternal diet and improved antenatal care leading to early detection and treatment of conditions such as diabetes, hypertension and anaemia. Specific advice on a high-folate diet to prevent neural-tube defects is important.

Perinatal factors

Improved obstetric care can prevent or reduce brain damage occurring at birth due to obstruction and hypoxia. An important contribution is made by early detection and treatment of babies who need additional support for hypoxia.

Postnatal factors and risks in early life

Preventive measures are directed at the various risk factors that may occur during development. Early detection and vigorous treatment of infections, and optimal management of chronic conditions such as epilepsy, hypothyroidism and phenylketonuria can significantly reduce the incidence and severity of disability. Accident prevention measures both within and outside the home, early detection and management of non-accidental injury and other forms of abuse and neglect, and stimulating environments have all been used with success.

Secondary prevention

Secondary prevention aims to treat or ameliorate the underlying condition in order to prevent or reduce disability. Examples include dietary regimes with a low phenylalanine content for individuals with phenylketonuria, and thyroxine replacement in neonates with congenital hypothyroidism.

Tertiary prevention

Tertiary prevention is aimed at minimising the sequelae of an existing disability. Examples include regular hearing, visual and thyroid checks for people with Down syndrome, and physiotherapy for children with cerebral palsy. Vigorous management of developmental delays in motor skills and communication can help to ameliorate the physical and psychological effects of under-stimulating home environments. Early diagnosis and appropriate treatment of coexisting epilepsy and psychiatric disorders will also reduce associated disabilities.

In a substantial majority of people with learning disabilities, it is difficult to establish a cause. A genetics laboratory will require information about which conditions are being considered, in order to run appropriate tests. For example, it is not currently possible to run broad genetic screens for any type of deletion – the laboratory will need to know which chromosome or chromosomes are likely to be affected. Clinical features of some of the commoner syndromes associated with learning disabilities are described in Chapter 6.

References

Department of Health Expert Advisory Group (1992) *Folic Acid and the Prevention of Neural Tube Defects*. Department of Health, London.

Gostason R, Wahlsrom J *et al.* (1991) Chromosomal aberrations in the mildly mentally retarded. *J Ment Defic Res.* **35:** 240–46.

McGuffin P (1994) *Seminars in Psychiatric Genetics.* Gaskell, London.

Sabaratnam M, Laver S, Butler L *et al.* (1994) Fragile X syndrome in North East Essex: towards systematic screening: clinical selection. *J Intellect Disabil Res.* **38:** 27–35.

Slaney SF, Wilkie AOM, Hirst MC *et al.* (1995) DNA testing for fragile X syndrome in schools for learning difficulties. *Arch Dis Child.* **72:** 33–7.

Further reading

McGuffin P (1994) *Seminars in Psychiatric Genetics.* Gaskell, London.

Part 2

Clinical aspects

This section considers the clinical features of disorders and conditions commonly associated with intellectual disability. It describes the causes, clinical presentations, classifications, frameworks for assessment and implications for the management of a variety of conditions such as psychiatric disorder, challenging behaviour, epilepsy, autism, and genetic and physical disorders. Disorders characteristic of childhood and adolescence and of old age are also described, and there is a section on aspects of sexuality in relation to people with an intellectual disability.

Chapter 3

Psychiatric disorders and challenging behaviour

David Clarke

Introduction

Learning disability is a condition characterised by significantly impaired cognitive functioning associated with problems with adaptive and social functioning, which becomes apparent before the age of 18 years. Psychiatric disorders are distinct from learning disabilities, and are characterised by abnormalities of emotional or behavioural functioning, relationships or thinking which are of a duration or severity that causes persistent suffering or handicap to the person concerned, or distress and disturbance to those in contact with him or her.

An individual can thus have both a learning disability and a psychiatric disorder. One consequence of having two conditions could be that the resulting disability is greater than if either of the disorders existed alone.

How common is psychiatric disorder?

Rutter *et al.* (1970) found that emotional and behaviour disorders were more common in children with intellectual retardation. They reported a fivefold increase in such disorders among children with nervous system disorders, such as cerebral palsy and epilepsy. Corbett (1979) surveyed children and adults with severe and profound learning disabilities and found that 47% of the children and 37% of the adults had a psychiatric disorder. Psychiatric disorders also occur more commonly in elderly people with learning disabilities than they do in the general elderly population (Cooper 1997).

Why are psychiatric disorders more common among people with learning disability?

The lifetime prevalence of severe psychiatric disorders among people with learning disabilities is about five times that among the general population. The reasons for the association are manifold, complex and interacting. Learning is a brain function, and both impaired learning and emotional and behavioural problems can result from brain damage or dysfunction. People with learning disability are also more vulnerable to adverse life events and psychosocial stressors that either predispose to or precipitate psychiatric illness. These include abuse, bullying, low self-esteem, loss and bereavement and physical illness. Physical problems such as infections or thyroid gland abnormalities can lead to psychiatric disorder, and epilepsy is associated with both learning disability and vulnerability to psychiatric disorders. Communication difficulties may compound a problem such as bereavement, making it more difficult to come to terms with grief. Some causes of learning disability are now known to be directly associated with a greatly increased risk of psychiatric disorder. Examples include Down syndrome and dementia, velocardiofacial syndrome and schizo-affective psychosis, and Prader–Willi syndrome caused by uniparental disomy and psychoses with affective symptoms (*see* Chapter 6 for further details).

Behaviour disorder or mental illness?

It is important to make a distinction between behaviour disorders and abnormal behaviours that are the result of an underlying mental illness. If problem behaviour is the manifestation of a mental illness (e.g. masturbating in public places as a symptom of a manic illness), it is less likely to respond to behavioural treatment and more likely to resolve after treatment of the underlying disorder.

Challenging behaviour

Behaviours that are problematic or challenging to services can arise for many reasons other than the presence of an underlying mental illness. People with learning disability may be bored or not engaged in activity that is meaningful to them. Their living environment may be noisy and crowded (this is likely to be particularly stressful for people who also have an autistic spectrum disorder). There may be difficulty obtaining attention from carers or communicating effectively with them. Problem behaviours may arise through attempts to communicate emotions such as misery or anxiety. Unusual or problematic behaviour may be the result of physical discomfort or pain. It may be a feature of an additional disability, such as the stereotyped rocking often associated with autism and the stereotyped hand wringing typical of Rett syndrome.

Behaviours that often lead to the involvement of psychiatric and psychological services for people with learning disability include aggressive behaviour, self-injury and property destruction. Fire-setting and abnormal sexual behaviour are relatively rare, and are likely to come to the attention of services because of the risks associated with them and the attendant likelihood of involvement of the criminal justice system.

Self-injury may have many different functions for one individual, and factors that initiate such behaviours (e.g. boredom) may be superseded by other changes (e.g. effects on neuromodulating compounds that alter pain sensation and mood). A knowledge of vulnerabilities associated with specific conditions (e.g. susceptibility to ear infections in people with Down syndrome and fragile X syndrome) allows the physical causes of challenging behaviours to be identified and dealt with, and a knowledge of the person's coping strategies and the characteristics of their environment (including the human environment) may identify psychological stressors.

The term 'challenging behaviour' is sometimes used to describe:

> behaviours of such an intensity, frequency or duration that the physical safety of the person or others is likely to be placed in serious jeopardy, or behaviour that is likely to seriously limit or delay access to or use of ordinary community facilities.

> (Emerson *et al.* 1987)

It is not a clinical diagnosis, but provision is made for it to be recorded in classificatory systems such as the ICD-10 and DC-LD (Royal College of Psychiatrists 2001). The onus is on professionals such as psychiatrists, psychologists and nurses to make accurate assessments and diagnoses and to help the person with a learning disability by reducing risks and maximising quality of life.

It is important that accurate diagnoses are made before treating any condition, and the diagnosis of psychiatric disorder in people with learning disabilities is no different. Diagnoses are helpful because they predict both responses to treatment and the prognosis. There are certain special issues that merit discussion here. Any illness can cause an impairment and may lead to disability. The person with a learning disability is already burdened with one. An undiagnosed and untreated mental illness will prevent the affected individual from achieving their potential. Consider the example of a man with moderate learning disabilities who is living at home with his parents and who shows periodic behaviour disturbance consisting of aggression, hyperactivity and poor sleep. If the recurrent mood disorder is not diagnosed and treated, he may end up being admitted to a hospital because his parents may be unable to cope. The disorder may also jeopardise his daytime activities and prevent him from going to the local shops, for example. Thus it will impact on his development and quality of life.

Diagnosis

The diagnosis of mental illness in people with learning disabilities can be problematic, especially if the diagnosis is one (such as schizophrenia) that depends on the communication of complex subjective experiences to the examining clinician. Language skills may be limited or absent, depending on the degree of disability that the individual has. People with mild learning disabilities are usually able to communicate how they feel, and it is possible to examine their thought processes. However, the assessment of whether a belief is truly delusional (i.e. false, held with conviction and not explicable on the basis of the person's cultural and educational background) may be difficult. People with learning disabilities may have false beliefs arising from misunderstanding, lack of community contact or the presence of an autistic disorder. Auditory hallucinations may be difficult to distinguish from practice vocalisations, conversations with (developmentally appropriate) invisible friends or stereotyped utterances associated with autism. Similar problems may arise with other phenomena such as thought disorder, and a high degree of language sophistication is necessary to describe passivity phenomena where, for example, the individual may feel that he or she is being controlled (Reid 1994). More often than not, family members and carers bring people with mild learning disabilities to appointments. It is important to obtain a corroborative history from them in order to gain a comprehensive picture of the difficulties. Another difficulty arises when the carer does not know the person with a learning disability well.

People with more severe learning disabilities and little communication present a different kind of challenge, because they may not be in a position to communicate about their inner world. In such cases a longitudinal history from a carer or family member who has known the individual well over a long period of time is crucial. Changes in sleep pattern, appetite, mood, self-help skills and sociability will provide valuable clues in the diagnosis of an underlying psychiatric condition, and it is often possible to establish diagnoses of mood disorders for people with such disabilities.

Psychiatrists usually rely on their skills in history taking and examination to reach a diagnosis of a mental illness. It may be necessary to see the individual on several occasions and in a variety of settings where they are more at ease, and to interview carers in both day and residential settings, interview family members and examine previous case notes before a diagnosis can be made. Rating scales such as the Leicester Kettering Depression Rating Scale and questionnaires such as the West Midlands Autism Questionnaire and Standardised Assessment of Personality Disorders can be used as adjuncts, as well as scales that are used in general adult psychiatry, such as the Hamilton Depression Rating Scale.

Moss *et al.* (1993) developed the Psychiatric Assessment Scale for Adults with Developmental Disability (PAS-ADD), which is derived from the Present State Examination (PSE) that was developed for use within general psychiatry. The Aberrant Behaviour Checklist (Aman *et al.* 1985) and the Diagnostic Assessment Scale for the Severely Handicapped (DASH) developed by Matson *et al.* (1991) were designed for use with people with severe learning disabilities, whereas the Reiss Screen for Maladaptive Behaviour (Reiss 1990) and the Psychopathology Inventory for Mentally Retarded Adults (PIMRA) (Matson *et al.* 1984) were developed for use with people with mild to moderate learning disabilities. These rating scales may be helpful either as research tools or to measure changes occurring during treatment.

Diagnoses of psychiatric disorders are based on the clinical guidelines contained in two classificatory systems. The *Diagnostic and Statistical Manual (DSM)* is the system used by the American Psychiatric Association, the latest version being DSM IV (American Psychiatric Association 1995). The World Health Organization published the tenth revision of the *International Classification of Diseases (ICD-10)* in 1992 (World Health Organization 1992). The latter is more commonly used in the UK. The World Health Organization later introduced the *ICD-10 Guide for Mental Retardation* ('mental retardation' being the commonest term used internationally to describe learning disabilities) (World Health Organization 1996). This guide was designed to enable those working in the field of learning disabilities to make the best use of the ICD-10. In 2001, the Royal College of Psychiatrists published the *Diagnostic Criteria for Psychiatric Disorders for Use with Adults with Learning Disabilities/Mental Retardation (DC-LD)*, which is used by psychiatrists in the UK.

Multi-axial diagnosis

People with learning disabilities usually have multiple problems. To describe these adequately it is usually necessary to use several diagnoses. The *ICD-10 Guide for Mental Retardation* (World Health Organization 1996) therefore recommends a

Table 3.1 System of diagnosis chart

Axis I	The severity of learning disabilities and problem behaviours
Axis II	Associated medical conditions (e.g. epilepsy, Down syndrome)
Axis III	Associated psychiatric disorders, including pervasive developmental disorders (e.g. autism)
Axis IV	Global assessment of psychosocial disability (using the WHO Short Disability Assessment Schedule)
Axis V	Associated abnormal psychosocial situations (e.g. institutional upbringing)

multi-axial system of diagnosis to record different types of features in the individual with learning disabilities. These axes are listed in Table 3.1 below.

Psychiatric disorders have been classified in many different ways, with most authors making a distinction between severe disorders (e.g. psychoses, in which reality testing is impaired) and less severe disorders. Psychoses may be symptomatic (e.g. the dementia accompanying Huntington's disease) or 'functional' (e.g. schizophrenia). The term 'functional' was originally used to describe psychotic disorders that were not associated with gross brain dysfunction. It continues to be used, in the absence of a more suitable term, despite evidence that disorders such as schizophrenia are associated with subtle changes in brain structure and function which are detectable using modern neuroimaging techniques. Terms used to describe symptoms of psychiatric illness include delusions (false beliefs that are held with absolute conviction, and that are not understandable, given the patient's social, educational and cultural background) and hallucinations (perceptions that occur without a stimulus). They are often auditory (heard), as in schizophrenia, or visual (seen), as in delirious states. It is useful to consider the different classes of mental illnesses and their presentation in people with learning disabilities.

Schizophrenia

Schizophrenia is characterised by fragmentation of thinking and by delusions and hallucinations of particular, often bizarre types. Schizophrenia literally means 'fragmented mind', and its popular use to describe a 'split personality' is incorrect. Schizophrenia may be the end result of more than one illness or process, and for this reason some clinicians prefer the collective term 'the schizophrenias'. Fragmentation of thought (often manifested as disordered speech, and sometimes manifested by the experience of having thoughts inserted into or withdrawn from the mind) is a key feature. Delusions of control or influence, or other bizarre delusions, specific types of auditory hallucinations, movement abnormalities and emotional abnormalities and disorders of the perception of free will may occur. Acts or emotions may be perceived as being made or imposed by some external agency ('passivity experiences'). Different types of schizophrenia are recognised, each with a characteristic pattern of symptoms and course. Schizophrenia is very rarely associated with dangerously aggressive behaviour towards other people. When this does occur in association with schizophrenia, the person concerned often has other problems such as substance abuse or a personality disorder.

The prevalence of schizophrenia is higher in the learning-disabled population (lifetime risk of around 3%) than in the general population (lifetime risk less than 1%). The prevalence among people with severe learning disabilities is impossible to ascertain because most of these individuals cannot describe the characteristic experiences (Reid 1994).

As the diagnosis of schizophrenia and related disorders may be difficult to establish, relatively non-specific categories (e.g. non-organic psychotic disorder) may have to be used. It may be difficult to differentiate between different subtypes of schizophrenia. The course of the disorder and the changes that occur over time should be taken into account. A decline in social, self-care or other skills and the development of unusual or apparently irrational maladaptive behaviour may be the earliest manifestation. Commonly reported symptoms include auditory hallucinations. Unexplained bizarre behaviours which are out of character and sustained in different environments should raise the possibility that the person may have delusions or hallucinations (World Health Organization 1996).

Mood disorders

Affective disorders or mood disorders are characterised by disturbances in mood and vitality, resulting in depression (with slowed thinking and impaired concentration, poor appetite, pessimism and ideas of guilt, self-reproach and self-harm) or elation (with euphoria, over-activity, talkativeness and ideas of grandiosity).

Depressive disorders are characterised by low mood, loss of interest or pleasure in activities that are normally pleasurable, early waking, worsening of low mood in the morning, reduction in activity and appetite, weight loss and reduction in libido. Depressive illness (or 'clinical depression') differs from everyday unhappiness or understandable low mood in that these additional features are present, although a depressive syndrome may be precipitated by an event (e.g. bereavement) that would be expected to cause unhappiness. Psychotic features such as delusions or hallucinations may accompany severe depressive episodes. Depressive disorders are associated with an increased risk of self-harm. This may take the form of suicide, or more commonly among people with learning disabilities, severely self-injurious behaviour or self-neglect. Affective disorders usually follow an episodic course, with years between episodes of illness (which usually last for a few months).

Manic and hypomanic states are characterised by elated mood (sustained for several days) accompanied by features such as overactivity, talkativeness, disinhibition, decreased need for sleep and distractibility. Mania is the more severe form of the disorder, and may be accompanied by delusions or hallucinations. Bipolar disorders are characterised by recurrent episodes of abnormal mood state, at least one of which has been manic or hypomanic.

Affective disorders (depression, manic-depressive illness and related conditions) are about five times more common among people with learning disabilities (both mild and severe) than in the general population, and the point prevalence in hospital studies is usually found to be around 2%.

Diagnosis may be hindered by the person's inability to communicate how he or she may be feeling. Disturbances in, for example, appetite, sleep pattern, interest in activities which give pleasure, self-help skills, sexual behaviour and level of arousal are useful indicators. Episodic self-injurious behaviour, screaming and withdrawal may often be diagnostic of mood disorders, functioning as depressive 'equivalents' (Marston *et al.* 1997).

Delirium and dementia

Dementias are characterised by progressive impairment of memory and other cognitive abilities, leading to impaired judgement and thinking. There is (at least initially) no reduction in the level of consciousness as seen in delirium, and other symptoms (e.g. emotional lability, irritability, apathy or coarsening of social behaviour) may be present. For a confident diagnosis to be made, symptoms should have been present for at least 6 months.

Delirium is characterised by a reduction in awareness of the environment ('clouded consciousness'), memory impairment, disorientation, changes in the pattern of activity (e.g. increased reaction time) and disturbance of the sleep–wake cycle.

Both dementia and delirium are characterised by disorientation (i.e. the person has a distorted sense of time, where they are, and who other people are), misinterpretation of the environment (e.g. imagining a bedroom to be a prison), and illusions or hallucinations – usually visual (e.g. seeing bodies fall past a window).

Dementia is associated with some specific causes of a learning disability, notably Down syndrome (Prasher 1993). Cooper (1997) found that the rate of dementia in older people with learning disabilities was four times higher than that in the general population. Other causes of cognitive deterioration, such as thyroid dysfunction and affective disorder masquerading as dementia, need to be ruled out. Longitudinal assessment of adaptive behaviours is a useful diagnostic tool.

Delirium may be the result of physical illness or intoxication. The risk of these disorders is increased among people with learning disabilities due to the presence of associated physical disorders and to drug treatments for problems such as epilepsy.

Neurotic, stress-related and somatoform disorders

These include phobias (i.e. fears of objects or situations), panic disorder (characterised by unpredictable, intense episodes of fear with an abrupt onset, lasting for minutes, and with features such as palpitations, sweating, or a feeling of 'going mad'), generalised anxiety, conversion ('hysterical') disorders and obsessive-compulsive disorder, which is characterised by obsessions (recurrent, unpleasant, intrusive thoughts that are resisted and which cause distress) or compulsions (actions that the person carries out repetitively while acknowledging that there is no reason for them to do so). Compulsive rituals may be difficult to distinguish from stereotyped activities which are usual among people with autism. A history of a change in behaviour, and the presence of resistance to the activity, may aid diagnosis. Some recent research suggests that rituals and stereotyped, repetitive behaviours may not be as distinct as was previously thought, and may share underlying biological mechanisms.

Some neuroses appear to be common in clinical practice, but this area has been less well researched than more severe disorders.

Eating disorders

Overeating and unusual dietary preferences are relatively common in people with learning disabilities, but eating disorders such as anorexia nervosa and bulimia are less frequent. The factors that are thought to contribute to these disorders, such as cultural expectations and societal pressures to be thin, may not have affected people with learning disabilities, who until recently were segregated in institutions. Perhaps they may become more common with the implementation of community care (World Health Organization 1996). Regurgitation, rumination and psychogenic vomiting are seen in people with learning disabilities.

Personality disorders

Personality disorders are deeply ingrained and enduring behaviour patterns that manifest themselves as inflexible responses to a broad range of personal and social situations. Such behaviour patterns tend to be stable and to encompass multiple domains of behaviour and psychological functioning (World Health Organization 1992).

Corbett (1979) reported a prevalence rate of around 25% for behaviour/personality disorder in his Camberwell study. The largest category consisted of people with impulsive or immature behaviour patterns. Khan *et al.* (1997) found that 31% of a community sample had a personality disorder.

These conditions are more easily diagnosed in people with mild learning disabilities, and the associated difficulties may result in contact with the criminal justice system.

Autism and related disorders

Autistic disorders, also called *pervasive developmental disorders* (PDDs), include childhood autism, atypical autism, Asperger's syndrome and some other categories. They are characterised by impairments in three areas.

1 Language may be delayed, abnormal or absent. The abnormalities may be gross, with muteness and no development of alternative means of communication (e.g. sign language), or subtle, with abnormal intonation, pedantic speech with a tendency to interpret remarks concretely, and inability to tailor speech to the social context.
2 Reciprocal social interactions are abnormal, with aloofness, solitariness or awkwardness in social situations, abnormalities of gaze, disinterest or distaste with regard to physical contact, and inability to 'play by the rules' in conversation.
3 There is a restricted, repetitive, stereotyped repertoire of interests and activities (e.g. collecting shiny objects or pieces of string, twirling or spinning objects, hand flapping), unusual fears or hobbies (e.g. collecting car registration numbers, memorising telephone numbers or bus routes, reciting varieties of

carrot), and insistence on predictability and familiarity, with intolerance of changes to routines, etc.

Autism and autistic spectrum disorders are discussed in Chapter 4.

Behavioural and psychiatric disorders with onset in childhood

These include hyperkinetic disorders, characterised by overactivity and deficits in attention, conduct and emotional disorders, and other disorders with an onset that is usually in childhood, such as enuresis (bed wetting), tics (sudden, involuntary, rapid, non-rhythmic, stereotyped movements or vocalisations) and Tourette's syndrome (combined vocal and multiple motor tics). Some of these disorders (e.g. hyperkinetic syndromes and tics) are not uncommon among people with learning disabilities, especially if the learning disability results from a genetic or metabolic abnormality.

Behavioural syndromes associated with particular disorders that cause learning disabilities are discussed further in Chapter 6.

Assessment and treatment

The last 30 years have seen the closure of learning disability hospitals and the introduction of care in the community for people with learning disabilities. These individuals are no longer considered by professionals and some others as people who should be hidden away from sight, and they are now encouraged to take their rightful place in society. This has meant that they are finally expected to use mainstream services, including health services, for their needs.

The expectation is that people with learning disabilities will consult general practitioners about their physical health problems and will be seen by appropriate hospital doctors if necessary. Psychiatrists in the field of learning disabilities no longer have responsibility for treating the physical problems of learning-disabled individuals, although they still sometimes have to advocate on behalf of their patients. However, it has been established that people with learning disabilities have higher rates of mental illness compared with the general population, and the presentation of such illness requires specific expertise, diagnosis and treatment. Therefore at the present time people with learning disabilities appear to need a specialised neuropsychiatric service, but with regard to treatment it should be emphasised that wherever possible people with learning disabilities should utilise the mainstream services used by the general population (Department of Health 2001). These issues are discussed further in Chapter 14.

When any treatment is provided, attention must be given to the likely benefits and the potential risks associated with it. No effective treatment (biological or psychological) is entirely free of potential unwanted effects. When prescribing for people whose ability to understand and communicate may be impaired, the tailoring of treatment to maximise potential gains and minimise adverse effects is especially important. This process requires a knowledge both of the treatment and its common adverse effects and of the problems to which the individual is vulnerable. For example, a man who has a schizophrenic illness and who is prone to constipation would be prescribed a different antipsychotic drug to a man who is prone to diarrhoea.

The effectiveness of drug treatments for severe psychiatric disorders has been established beyond doubt, but the treatment of many 'challenging' behaviours associated with learning disabilities is empirically based (Clarke 1997). This is partly a result of methodological problems with clinical trials (e.g. ensuring that there are adequate numbers of people with the same psychiatric disorder and the same cause and severity of learning disability). Many reports in the literature describe the treatment of small numbers of people with learning disability, or single cases. The results often imply that some, but not most, people with a particular problem will benefit from the treatment. Clinicians are therefore usually more cautious when using drugs to treat such disorders, because the risks remain but the benefits may not be so clearly established.

The drugs used to treat mental illness in people with learning disabilities are no different from those used in the general population. The *British National Formulary* guides the psychiatrist on dosage and side-effects. Schizophrenia, mania and other psychotic disorders are treated with antipsychotic drugs. Chlorpromazine, trifluoperazine, thioridazine and haloperidol are older drugs with more side-effects. As in general psychiatry, the trend is to use newer, 'cleaner' drugs such as risperidone. Zuclopenthixol appears to be effective in people who are aggressive.

For patients who present with a depressive illness, again the trend is to use the newer antidepressants such as the selective serotonin reuptake inhibitors (e.g. paroxetine), as they cause fewer side-effects. This is particularly important as these patients may be on other drugs such as anticonvulsants. Lithium and carbamazepine are used as mood stabilisers in individuals with bipolar affective disorders. Liquid preparations of medication are useful, as sometimes patients may either chew tablets or find it difficult to swallow them. Depot preparations of antipsychotic drugs are useful in cases where compliance may not be guaranteed. Electroconvulsive therapy is only rarely used in people with learning disabilities.

When a person with a learning disability has an additional mental illness, medication will only be one aspect of the treatment. The psychiatrist specialising in learning disabilities is a member of a multi-disciplinary team, and other professionals will make important contributions to ensure the patient's well-being. These issues are discussed further in Chapters 13 and 14.

References

Aman MG, Singh NN, Stewart AW *et al.* (1985) The Aberrant Behaviour Checklist: a behaviour rating scale for the assessment of treatment effects. *Am J Ment Defic.* **89:** 485–91.

American Psychiatric Association (1995) *Diagnostic and Statistical Manual of Mental Disorders* (4e) *(DSM-IV, International Version).* American Psychiatric Association, Washington, DC.

Clarke DJ (1997) Towards rational psychotropic prescribing for people with learning disability. *Br J Learn Disabil.* **25:** 46–52.

Cooper S-A (1997) Learning disabilities and old age. *Adv Psychiatr Treat.* **3:** 312–20.

Corbett JA (1979) Psychiatric morbidity and mental retardation. In: FE James and RP Snaith (eds) *Psychiatric Illness and Mental Handicap.* Gaskell, London.

Department of Health (2001) *Valuing People: a new strategy for learning disability for the twenty-first century.* The Stationery Office, London.

Emerson E, Barrett S, Bell C *et al.* (1987) *Developing Services for People with Severe Learning Difficulties and Challenging Behaviours.* Institute of Social and Applied Psychology, Canterbury.

Khan A, Cowan C and Roy A (1997) Personality disorders in people with learning disabilities: a community survey. *J Intellect Disabil Res.* **41:** 324–30.

Marston GM, Perry DW and Roy A (1997) Manifestations of depression in people with intellectual disability. *J Intellect Disabil Res.* **41:** 476–80.

Matson JL, Kazdih AE and Senatore V (1984) Psychometric properties of the psychopathology instrument for mentally retarded adults. *Appl Res Ment Retard.* **5:** 881–9.

Matson JL, Gardner WI, Coe DA *et al.* (1991) A scale for evaluating emotional disorders in severely and profoundly mentally retarded persons: development of the Diagnostic Assessment for the Severely Handicapped (DASH) Scale. *Br J Psychiatry.* **159:** 404–9.

Moss S, Patel P, Prosser H *et al.* (1993) Psychiatric morbidity in older people with moderate and severe learning disability. 1. Development and reliability of the Patient Interview (PAS-ADD). *Br J Psychiatry.* **163:** 471–80.

Prasher VP (1993) Down's syndrome, longevity and Alzheimer's disease. *Br J Psychiatry.* **162:** 710.

Reid AH (1994) Psychiatry and learning disability. *Br J Psychiatry.* **164:** 613–18.

Reiss S (1990) Prevalence of dual diagnosis in community-based day programmes in the Chicago Metropolitan Area. *Am J Ment Retard.* **94:** 578–85.

Royal College of Psychiatrists (2001) *Diagnostic Criteria for Psychiatric Disorders for Use with Adults with Learning Disabilities/Mental Retardation (DC-LD)*. Gaskell, London.

Rutter ML, Tizard J and Whitmore K (eds) (1970) *Education, Health and Behaviour*. Longman, London.

World Health Organization (1992) *The ICD-10 Classification of Mental and Behavioural Disorders: clinical descriptions and diagnostic guidelines*. World Health Organization, Geneva.

World Health Organization (1996) *ICD-10 Guide for Mental Retardation*. World Health Organization, Geneva.

Chapter 4

Autism and other developmental disorders

Meera Roy

Introduction

Autism belongs to a group of conditions known as *pervasive developmental disorders*, which are characterised by qualitative abnormalities in reciprocal social interactions and patterns of communication, and by a restricted stereotyped repetitive repertoire of interests and activities (ICD-10) (World Health Organization 1992). These qualitative abnormalities are a pervasive feature of the individual's functioning in all situations.

In 1943, Leo Kanner described a group of children who had in common an unusual pattern of behaviour which he termed 'infantile autism'. They had a profound lack of affective contact, intense insistence on sameness in their self-chosen, often bizarre and elaborate repetitive routines, muteness or marked abnormality of speech, fascination with and ability in manipulating objects, and good visuospatial skill in contrast with learning difficulties in other areas. In 1944, Hans Asperger described children with a cluster of behaviours which now bear the name *Asperger's syndrome*. These young people were naive in their social interactions, had intense circumscribed interests, good grammar and vocabulary but monotonous speech, poor motor ability, marked lack of common sense and specific learning disabilities. Asperger admitted that there were similarities between the syndrome that he had described and that described by Leo Kanner.

The concept of autism has evolved over the years, and it is now recognised that the spectrum ranges from people with severe learning disabilities at one end to somewhat eccentric individuals at the other. Common to all people with autistic disorders is the triad of impairments described by Lorna Wing and Judith Gould, which consists of impairments in social interactions and social communication, and repetitive stereotyped patterns of behaviours and interests.

The condition existed long before it was first described by Leo Kanner. Lorna Wing, in her book *The Autistic Spectrum* (Wing 1996), describes various historical figures who may have had an autistic disorder. Brother Juniper, an early follower of St Francis, had a complete inability to understand social situations, and when the citizens of Rome came to welcome him he ignored them as a seesaw caught his attention. Victor, the 'wild boy' of Aveyron described by Itard, behaved like a child with autism. Other notable figures who may have had an autistic condition include Albert Einstein, Sir Isaac Newton and Henry Cavendish.

Classification

Autism and related conditions are grouped under pervasive developmental disorders in both the *ICD-10 Classification of Mental and Behavioural Disorders* (World Health Organization 1992) and the revised fourth edition of the *Diagnostic and Statistical Manual of Mental Disorders (DSM-IV-R)* (American Psychiatric Association 2000). Childhood autism is defined as abnormal or impaired development that is manifested before the age of 3 years, with abnormal functioning in reciprocal social interactions, communication and restricted stereotyped repetitive behaviours. Atypical autism differs either in age of onset or in failure to fulfil all three sets of diagnostic criteria. Rett's syndrome (usually found in girls) is included in this group, although a specific genetic abnormality of MECP2 has been established. Asperger's syndrome differs from childhood autism in that there is no general delay in language or cognitive development. *ICD-10* also includes other childhood disintegrative disorders and overactivity disorder associated with mental retardation and stereotyped movements. Both DSM-IV-R and ICD-10 have a category of *pervasive developmental disorder unspecified*.

Prevalence

The definition of autistic disorder has evolved from Leo Kanner's definition to the concept of spectrum with the *triad of impairments*, and the prevalence has changed with the definition. In 1966, Lotter reported a prevalence of 4.1 in 10 000 for autism in Middlesex. However, more recent surveys suggest that the prevalence for all forms of pervasive developmental disorder may be as high as 60 in 10 000 (Fombonne 2003). Autism is associated with learning disability in about 70% of cases, and is over-represented in males, with a male:female ratio of 4.3:1. It is also found in association with some rare and genetically determined medical conditions such as tuberous sclerosis. People with conditions such as Smith–Magenis syndrome and fragile X syndrome show a behavioural syndrome that overlaps with the autistic syndrome.

Clinical features

The triad of impairments forms the core of autistic disorders. As mentioned above, these are:

1 impairment in social interactions
2 impairment in social communication
3 restricted, stereotyped activities and interests.

People on the autistic spectrum also have impairments in imagination, which can be included under either social communication or repetitive behaviours.

   Autistic disorders are dimensional rather than categorical disorders, and when making the diagnosis it is important to take into account the disability due to the impairments. A person with the triad of impairments may not show any disability at all, as they may have adequate support mechanisms and be in an environment where their profiles are an advantage. As long as an individual is comfortable where they are, there is no need for a diagnosis.

Impairment in social interactions

People with autistic conditions often have difficulties making friends and prefer to be on their own. They avoid doing things with other people and do not feel the need to share their interests and achievements with others. Parents of children with autism often comment that they did not know of their child's achievement until they met the teacher at school. Autistic individuals have difficulty identifying how other people feel, either not recognising their emotions at all or misreading them. Even when they recognise another person's mood state they are not able to show appropriate responses. For example, consider the child with autism who when told that his carer is ill either shows no response at all or is upset that there may be no one to take him to his weekly swimming session. People with autistic conditions have difficulties in using their own body language to regulate social interactions. This could include the use of gaze (either staring or not making eye contact at all) and the use of facial expressions, body posture and gestures.

The impairments in social interactions also span a spectrum, and in her book *The Autistic Spectrum*, Lorna Wing has described three groups of presentations, namely aloof, passive, and active but odd.

The aloof group

These people seem to be cut off and in a world of their own, and behave as if other people do not exist. Their faces may be empty of expression and they have no interest in or sympathy for others. They tend to use other people as objects for their use.

The passive group

These people are not totally cut off from others, and are likely to make eye contact when reminded to do so. As they are amenable and willing, other children often involve them in play in childhood. They accept social approaches and do not move away from others, but they do not initiate social interactions.

The active but odd group

This group presents a considerable challenge with regard to diagnosis. They make active approaches in a peculiar one-sided fashion to make their demands. They pay little attention to the feelings of other people, and often stare too long and hard. Their physical approaches can be intrusive and can become immediately aggressive.

Impairment in social communication

People with autism have difficulties in both communication and language. Speech often develops late, and there may be abnormalities such as echolalia (where words are repeated), delayed echolalia (where dialogues from television programmes may be repeated verbatim), pronominal reversal (where 'you' is used in the place of 'I') and repetition of words and phrases. Some people do not develop speech at all and may also have difficulty using non-verbal means of communication. They also show unusual modulation of speech, which can be very loud or very soft and may be monotonous. Their speech may be telegraphic, leaving out connecting words such as 'and' and 'is'.

People with autism may have difficulty understanding that words may have different meanings in different contexts, and that words which sound the same may be spelt differently and mean different things. They can be literal in their understanding, which may make it difficult for them to understand jokes and sarcasm. They may use words in a different context to their usual meaning, and they may make up new words. They thus show both semantic and pragmatic difficulties in their speech. Some develop speech at about the usual age or even ahead of other children, and appear to have a fascination with words. They may be formal in their speech and pedantic in the use of words. This is more commonly seen in people with Asperger's syndrome or high-functioning autism. Although they may have adequate speech production, their under-standing may be at a much lower level.

People with autistic disorders may have difficulty in taking turns in conversa-tion, not knowing how to start and finish an interaction. They may be abrupt and interrupt frequently, or they may not say anything at all. People with autistic syndromes often have difficulties with make-believe and pretending. They are not good at lying, and when they do lie it is very obvious.

Sometimes the impairments in communication are very marked, obscuring the other impairments, and the individual may be given a diagnosis of *semantic pragmatic disorder*. However, the other difficulties coexist and need to be identified if the person is to be appropriately supported.

Repetitive patterns of behaviours and interests

People with autistic disorders often spend long periods of time absorbed in their special interests at the expense of other necessary activities. These interests may include collecting facts about cars and aircraft, studying encyclopaedias, bus routes or timetables, or watching certain television programmes or videos. They may be upset when they are unable to carry out these activities. They like to have a routine and can be distressed by any change. This may include the order in which they get ready in the mornings or the route to school. They may engage in rituals such as the lining up of toy cars or ornaments.

Adults and children with autistic disorders are often interested in the feel, taste or smell of materials. They may want to study objects from different angles or look at the pattern of light and shadows. They may display repetitive body movements such as rocking, spinning, flapping of the hands, flicking of the fingers or flicking bits of string. These behaviours indicate unusual sensory preferences as a result of abnormal multi-sensory integration. They may be hyper- or hyposensitive to different sensation.

Hypersensitivity to sounds may lead children with autism to cover their ears. Often there is hyposensitivity to pain, so that people with autism may pick at sores, reopen wounds or not report pain due to injuries. There may also be abnormalities in cross-modal integration of sensations, leading to synaesthesia with difficulty in distinguishing between various sensory inputs.

Onset and course

Autism has its beginnings in infancy. Some children begin to develop normally and then lose skills, while others show late development. They are usually symptomatic by the age of three years. A detailed history often shows difficulties in social interactions as early as the first year. The baby may be difficult to comfort and may not like being cuddled. Some babies may also be described as being very good because they do not demand social attention. They may be late in developing joint attention, such as pointing things out to parents. As they do not like change there may be difficulties with weaning to solid foods and with toilet training. Playgroups and nursery present a challenge, as these children may be solitary and find it difficult to play with others and make friends. Such difficulties continue into school, where these children may be bullied.

Speech development merits special consideration. This is often delayed, and there may be a need for speech therapy. Some children do not develop speech at all, and this is associated with significant degrees of learning disability. Children who are given a diagnosis of Asperger's syndrome do not show cognitive impairment, and they develop speech normally or even early. They may be pedantic and like to use unusual words. An example is that of a three-year-old who asked his mother not to be 'a nincompoop'. Some children who have had speech delay and speech therapy may grow up to have a speech repertoire similar to that of individuals with a diagnosis of Asperger's syndrome.

Coexisting conditions

Children with autism also seem to display features of hyperactivity. Although both *DSM-IV* and *ICD-10* state that when autism is already present, hyperactivity is not diagnosed separately, the latter compounds the disability and merits treatment.

Some children with autism have difficulty with fine motor coordination and can present as clumsy children who may receive a diagnosis of dyspraxia. Christopher Gillberg (2003) found that among children with disorders of attention, motor coordination and perception (referred to as DAMP syndrome) there are a number of cases with autistic disorders.

People with autistic conditions often have high levels of anxiety, and the incidence of mood disorders also seems to be higher in these individuals.

What causes autism?

The majority of epidemiological surveys have ruled out social class as a risk factor for autism, and there is a lack of variation in the incidence according to race or ethnicity (Fombonne 2003). When Kanner first described autism, psychoanalytical theories were popular and autism was considered to be an emotional disorder brought about by the way in which parents brought up their children. Fortunately, later research has established that autism is a developmental disorder.

It is not known whether autism is a single syndrome with variable severity or an aggregate of specific disorders that share common features. What seems clear, however, is that there are multiple aetiologies. It is possible that dysfunction of certain brain areas or networks could produce reasonably predictable behavioural deficits, and in autism this could be the result of genetic and environmental factors expressed morphologically as alterations in early brain development (Acosta and Pearl 2003).

Genetic studies

Twin and family studies show significant differences in monozygotic compared with dizygotic concordance rates, suggesting an underlying genetic predisposition. The rate of autism in siblings of a person with autism is higher than in the general population, indicating the involvement of multiple susceptibility genes. Genome-wide linkage analyses of families with autism have yielded positive signals for chromosomes 1, 2q, 7q, 9, 13, 15q, 16p, 17q, 19, 22 and X, with 2q and 7q appearing to be the best candidate regions for containing an autism locus. The FOXP2 gene linked to speech–language disorder 1, and the RELN gene, a candidate gene for autism which codes for reelin, are both associated with chromosome 7.

A proportion of autistic individuals have known genetic conditions such as tuberous sclerosis, neurofibromatosis and fragile X syndrome. Cytogenetic screening for chromosomal abnormalities shows that chromosome 15 and X-chromosome break points are most frequently associated with autism. GABA receptor gene polymorphisms and the UBE3A, an Angelman syndrome gene at the critical area on chromosome 15, have been associated with autism.

Neuroimaging studies: growth dysregulation hypothesis

Abnormalities have been reported in specific brain regions, including the cerebellum and temporal lobe. Recent magnetic resonance imaging (MRI) studies suggest that there is abnormal brain growth in autism, with early overgrowth followed by abnormally slow growth in some regions and premature arrest in others. The abnormal growth pattern may also include a lack of acceleration in adolescence usually associated with the emergence of a second phase of higher-order abilities, including frontal lobe functions. Nelson *et al.* (2001) found elevated levels of brain neurotrophins and neuropeptides in neonatal blood spots of individuals who later developed autism and mental retardation. These and other growth factors play an important role in neuronal proliferation, migration, differentiation, growth and circuit organisation. Such elevated levels may form the molecular basis for the early acceleration in brain growth.

Neuropathological studies

Gross neuropathological abnormalities are not typical in autism, but abnormalities at the cellular level have been observed. These include curtailed development of neurons in the forebrain limbic system, a congenital decrease in the number of Purkinje cells in the cerebellum, and age-related differences in cell size and neuronal number in the cerebellar nuclei and inferior olivary nucleus of the brainstem (Kemper and Bauman 1998).

The minicolumn is the fundamental anatomical and physiological unit of vertical organisation in the cerebral cortex. In the adult brain the minicolumns appear as thin radial structures ranging from 30 to 60 microns in width depending on the cortical area. Each minicolumn contains a repetitive array of afferent input from the thalamus, intrinsic microcircuitry and efferent output, endowing the structure with a putative role as a physiological unit (Casanova *et al.* 2002). The minicolumns are separated by peripheral neuropil space containing dendritic arborisations, synapses and unmyelinated axons. The cells also exert lateral inhibition to sharpen borders and increase definition. In autism, more numerous, smaller and less compact minicolumns have been described, which suggests that there may be more processing units per unit of brain surface without a corresponding increase in the number of thalamic afferents. The failure to assimilate extra processing units may result in cortical 'noise', which then overtaxes the system.

Autism has been regarded as a disorder of the arousal-modulating system of the brain. Autistic individuals experience a chronic state of over-arousal and exhibit abnormal behaviours. An increase in the number of minicolumns and impairment of the inhibitory GABA-ergic neurons that maintain the lateral inhibition in the minicolumns would alter the connective patterns between thalamic input and cerebral cortex, and would affect the ability to discriminate between competing types of sensory information.

Fatemi *et al.* (2001) reported dysregulation of the proteins reelin (a signalling protein that guides neuronal migration in the fetus and is involved in the cellular signalling system which subserves cognition in the adult brain) and Bcl-2 (which governs programmed cell death), with a reduction of both proteins in autistic cerebellar tissue compared with control samples. This reduction may explain the abnormalities in autism.

Neurotransmitter studies and serotonergic dysregulation

Serotonin is known to play a role in brain development prior to the time when it assumes its function as a neurotransmitter in the mature brain. It regulates both the development of serotonergic neurons (termed autoregulation of development) and the development of target tissues (Whitaker-Azmitia 2001). It influences the processes of neurogenesis, neuronal differentiation, neuropil formation, axon myelination and synaptogenesis. Removal of serotonin early in development in rats causes a permanent reduction in the number of neurons in the adult brain in hippocampus and cortex. At a later stage in development, serotonin plays a role in dendritic development, including overall dendritic length, spine formation and branching both in the hippocampus and in the cortex. However, as the animal reaches the early weaning stage and serotonin levels should be declining, excess serotonin levels seem to 'arrest' spine development. In adult animals, removal of serotonin causes loss of dendrites. Serotonin levels can be affected by multiple and non-specific postnatal factors including hypoxia, viral infections, malnutrition, social enrichment and stress. Drugs such as cocaine, nicotine and alcohol can alter serotonin levels.

Increasing evidence points to an imbalance in serotonin levels as a possible factor in the aetiology of autism. Both an abundance and a paucity of serotonin may be deleterious. Depletion of serotonin levels results in a significant delay in maturation of the somatosensory cortex in rats, while excessive levels early in development result in hyperinnervation and expansion of cortical structure, and may contribute to an increase in the number of minicolumns.

Comparative studies on monoamine levels in children with autism and controls suggest that there is abnormal maturation of the serotonergic system during development.

Cognitive theories

The three cognitive theories of autism are mind blindness and impaired theory of mind, the weak central coherence theory and the executive dysfunction theory.

Mind blindness and impaired theory of mind

In 1984 Nicholas Humphrey said that human beings are 'born psychologists'. The ability to read other people's intentions and to interpret behaviours in terms of a person's mental state is inborn, and is the result of a long process of evolution. Infants watch movement and learn to look where their caregivers look. They look when objects are pointed out to them, and later they begin to point out things themselves. By the end of the first year of life, normal infants can tell that they and someone else are attending to the same thing, and they can read other people's actions as goal-directed and driven by desires. As toddlers they can pretend and understand pretence. By the time they start school at around the age of 4 years, they can work out what people might think, know and believe. This ability may be impaired in people with autism, so that they have difficulties in reading other people to the extent that they are 'mind blind' (Baron-Cohen 1997).

Baron-Cohen has shown that such mind blindness may be due to impairments in the 'theory of mind mechanism'. This consists of representing mental states which include pretending, thinking, knowing, believing, imagining, dreaming, guessing and deceiving, and linking together these mental state concepts into a coherent understanding of how mental state and actions are related.

The Sally Ann test is a demonstration of theory of mind mechanisms, and it has been used in children with autism or Down syndrome and in normal children. It involves Sally putting a marble in one place and going away. While she is away Ann puts the marble somewhere else. The child needs to appreciate that since Sally was absent when the marble was moved she must believe that it is still in the original location. In response to the test question 'Where will Sally look for the marble?', the vast majority of normal children and those with Down syndrome passed, indicating the original location of the marble, whereas only a small minority of the children with autism did so. Instead, most of them indicated where the marble really was. The test is illustrated in Figure 4.1.

In imaging studies, autistic people show weak activation of the medial prefrontal cortex and superior temporal gyrus when performing theory of mind tasks. This and the failure to activate the 'fusiform face area' during face perception tasks may stem from a lack of integration of sensory processing with cognitive evaluation. This may be a result of brain maturation abnormalities, abnormal connectivity and lack of pruning (Frith 2003).

Weak central coherence theory

This relates to the difficulty that people with autism have in seeing the whole, because they tend to focus on detail. The weak central coherence leads to problems in making sense of perceptions and thus to difficulties in communication, and has been seen as a crucial deficit in autism.

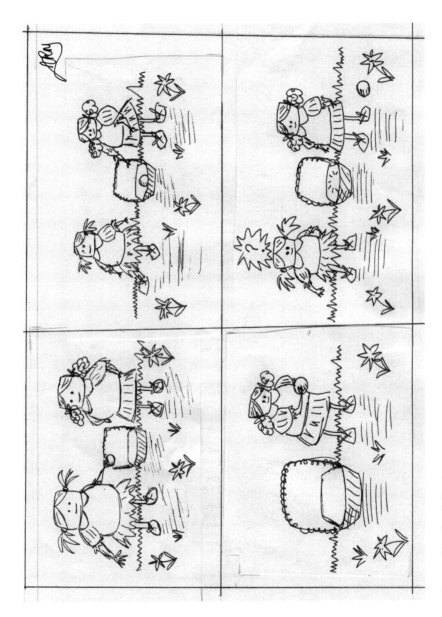

Figure 4.1 The Sally Ann test.

Executive dysfunction theory

One of the most consistently replicated cognitive deficits in people with autism is executive dysfunction. Executive functions include the many skills required to prepare for and execute complex behaviour, including planning, inhibition organisation, self-monitoring, mental representation of tasks and goals, cognitive flexibility and set shifting. Executive functions are thought to be driven by the prefrontal cortex (Duncan 1986). Imaging, neuropathological and neuropsychological studies indicate that the frontal cortex is involved in autism. A recent study indicated that people with autism had deficits in planning efficiency and extra dimensional shifting compared with controls, which was correlated with their adaptive behaviour (Ozonoff *et al.* 2004).

Extreme male brain

Baron-Cohen and colleagues have divided the human brain into two types, namely the empathising brain, which is better at empathising and communicating and is more common in women, and the systemising brain, which is better at understanding and building systems, and is more common in men. People with autism are weaker with regard to communication and empathy and are stronger on systemising tasks. Baron-Cohen has suggested that autism is an example of the extreme male brain (Baron-Cohen 2003).

Diagnosis

The diagnosis of autism is a clinical one and is made by taking a detailed developmental history from the parents and by assessment of the individual. Both *DSM-IV* and *ICD-10* set out criteria by which a diagnosis may be made. A child who displays unusual social behaviours may initially be screened by the health visitor or general practitioner using the Checklist for Autism in Toddlers (CHAT) or the Childhood Autism Rating Scale, which can lead to a more detailed clinical assessment.

There are various screening tools available, such as the Social Communication questionnaire (SCQ), the Pervasive Developmental Disorder Mental Retardation Scale (PDD-MRS) and the Developmental Behaviour Checklist (DBC), which can be used to screen groups of people for autistic conditions. In addition, there are observation schedules such as the Autism Diagnostic Observation Schedule (ADOS), the Autism Diagnostic Interview (ADI) and the Diagnostic Interview for Social and Communication Disorders (DISCO), which can be used to conduct systematic assessments.

Baron-Cohen and his colleagues have devised a series of questionnaires looking at empathy and systemising quotients and autism quotients, which can help to reach a diagnosis in cases of Asperger's syndrome and in people with higher-functioning autism.

Management

Because autism is a developmental disorder rather than an illness, the focus of interventions is to help the individual to function adaptively. The first step is early diagnosis, and in the UK most children are diagnosed by community paedia-tricians. Parents will usually have been concerned that their child is somewhat different, and may have initiated the process. There may be a need for speech and language therapy interventions in the event of delayed speech, and the child may also be offered a place at a specialist nursery. Assessment at a Child Development Centre would include screening for any dyspraxia, and there may be interven-tions undertaken by occupational therapists.

The child may receive a statement of special educational need and may be supported in mainstream education, or they may be placed in a specialist school. Senior school years present particular challenges to children on the autistic spectrum, and it is important for the support to continue. Many colleges of further education offer provision for people on the autistic spectrum. The Disabled Student Allowance provides further support for students to access university courses. Autistic disorders are accepted as a disability, and there may be entitlement to the Disability Living Allowance. Autism is a lifelong condition, and the need for support will vary depending on what else is going on in the individual's life.

In the UK, the National Autistic Society is a resource for people with autism and their families. There are also regional societies that offer support, training and accommodation.

A person with autism may find it difficult to fit into existing educational approaches, and the system may have to be modified to meet the autistic person's needs. Approaches such as TEACCH (Treatment and Education of Autistic and related Communication Handicapped Children) focus on the strengths and interests of the individual and engage them.

The thrust of interventions is educational and social. However, comorbid conditions may require treatment. Hyperarousal and anxiety can be disabling, and must be reduced in order to enable the person to engage. Engagement in small groups with support, noise reduction and the use of visual cues can be helpful. A sensory assessment may identify hypo- and hypersensitive sensory inputs which can be manipulated to relax the individual. Low doses of neuro-leptics, particularly risperidone, appear to reduce anxiety. Drugs that increase serotonergic activity seem to have an effect in reducing repetitive behaviours.

Up to 30% of children with autism also appear to meet the criteria for the diagnosis of attention deficit hyperactivity disorder (ADHD). These children benefit from having the condition treated. Their response to stimulant medication is not as good as that in children without autism, but it is important to treat the ADHD in a systematic way.

A significant number of people with autism develop epilepsy, which will need to be treated.

People with autistic conditions appear to be more at risk of developing mood disorders compared with the general population. At times of stress they are also likely to develop psychotic episodes, which may be mistaken for schizophrenia. It is important to distinguish between the two conditions, as the treatment and prognosis are different.

Hyperkinetic disorders

These consist of a group of disorders with onset in childhood, no later than 7 years of age, nearly always before the age of 5 years and frequently before the age of 2 years (Taylor *et al.* 2004). Affected children show a lack of persistence in activities that require cognitive involvement, a tendency to shift from task to task without completing any of them, and disorganised ill-regulated activity that is pervasive across different situations, persistent over time and not caused by other disorders such as autism or affective disorders. The affected individuals show clinically significant impairment of social, academic or occupational functioning. These disorders often persist into adolescence and adult life, and put the person at risk of adverse outcomes such as delinquency, antisocial behaviour and underachievement.

The diagnostic criteria set out in *ICD-10* for hyperkinetic disorder and in *DSM-IV-R* for attention deficit disorder/hyperactivity are similar, although the latter is more broadly defined. In both schemes the three problems of attention, hyperactivity and impulsivity are to be recognised. In *ICD-10* all three should be present and should be pervasive across situations. However, *ICD-10* also recognises sub-threshold conditions such as attention deficit disorder, activity disorder, and home-specific and classroom-specific disorders. The groups in *DSM-IV-R* are ADHD combined, predominantly inattentive, predominantly hyperactive–impulsive and NOS (not otherwise specified). In the rest of this discussion the terms hyperactivity disorder and ADHD will be used interchangeably.

The prevalence of hyperkinetic disorders is 3–5%, with a male preponderance. Hyperkinetic disorders are seen in people with all levels of IQ and in all socio-economic classes. ADHD aggregates within families, with a three- to fivefold increased risk in first-degree relatives (Faraone and Biederman 1994). Twin studies indicate considerable heritability, with genetic factors contributing 65–90% of the phenotypic variance in the population (Thapar *et al.* 1999).

Boys tend to present with hyperactivity earlier, while girls may present later, at 14 or 15 years of age, with inattention. Hyperactive–impulsive symptoms tend to decline over time while inattentive symptoms persist. In girls and women, symptoms may become more prominent at menarche and menopause.

What causes hyperkinetic disorders?

Structural and functional brain imaging studies implicate catecholamine-rich fronto-subcortical pathways in the pathophysiology of ADHD (Biederman and Faraone 2002). There is evidence of decreased dopaminergic activity in the mesocortical and mesolimbic pathways in ADHD. The altered activity in the mesocortical pathways may lead to impairment of frontal executive functions, so that people with ADHD have difficulty organising and prioritising, shifting and sustaining attention, regulating alertness, effort and processing speed, managing frustration, using working memory and monitoring and self-regulating action. The involvement of the reward circuits of the mesolimbic pathways may lead to intolerance of delay and delay aversion (Sonuga-Barke 2002).

The dopaminergic system, and in particular the dopamine D_2 receptor, has been implicated in reward mechanisms. The net effect of neurotransmitter interaction at the mesolimbic brain region induces a 'reward' when dopamine is released from the neuron at the nucleus accumbens and interacts with a dopamine D_2 receptor. The 'reward cascade' involves the release of serotonin, which in turn at the hypothalamus stimulates enkephalin, which then inhibits GABA at the substantia nigra, which in turn fine tunes the amount of dopamine released at the nucleus accumbens or 'reward site.' It is well known that under normal conditions in the reward site dopamine works to maintain our normal drives. In fact, dopamine has come to be known as the 'pleasure molecule' and/or the 'anti-stress molecule.' When dopamine is released into the synapse, it stimulates a number of receptors (D_1 to D_5), which results in increased feelings of well-being and stress reduction. A consensus of the literature suggests that when there is dysfunction in the brain reward cascade, which could be caused by certain genetic variants (polygenic), especially in the dopaminergic system (causing a hypodo-paminergic trait), the brain of that person requires a dopamine 'fix' in order to feel good. Blum *et al.* (2000) coined the term *reward deficiency syndrome* to describe this hypodopaminergic state.

Alcohol, cocaine, heroin, marijuana, nicotine and glucose all cause activation and neuronal release of brain dopamine, which could heal the abnormal cravings. A hypodopaminergic state could thus lead to addictive behaviour, and people with ADHD can have substance abuse as the presenting symptom. Exercise and risk-taking behaviour increase dopamine release through the release of cortico-trophin-releasing hormone.

People with the A1 allele of the D_2-receptor gene appear to have lower levels of the D_2 receptor and an increased risk of addiction. A variant of the D_4-receptor gene has been associated with novelty-seeking behaviours. Abnormalities have also been seen in the dopamine-transporter gene, with its activity decreasing with age. Each of these risk alleles increases the relative risk for ADHD only slightly, showing that the latter is a complex disorder influenced by the interaction of multiple aetiological factors, each of which has a minor effect. It has also been suggested that ADHD and reading ability and also ADHD and autism share genetic susceptibility factors (Taylor *et al.* 2004).

There are associations with a variety of environmental risks, including prenatal and perinatal obstetric complications, low birth weight, prenatal exposure to benzodiazepines, alcohol or nicotine, and brain disease and injury. Severe early deprivation, institutional rearing, idiosyncratic reactions to food and exposure to lead are also considered to be risk factors. The quality of relationships within the family and at school may have either maintaining or protective effects.

ADHD appears to represent a heterogeneous group of dysfunctions, and there may be multiple developmental pathways from aetiological factors to behav-ioural symptoms. The diagnosis of ADHD is a dimensional one. Everyone sometimes shows some impairment in executive functions, but in people with ADHD it is chronic and causes severe impairment. The symptoms can show situational variability, and for most people with the condition there are some activities where the impairment is absent. This is particularly well illustrated by children who can concentrate on their computer games but not on their homework. They are able to concentrate on things that interest them, and computer games offer an immediate reward. On the other hand, people who are not impaired by hyperactivity can make themselves do things in which they are not interested.

Comorbidity

Children with hyperkinetic disorders are more likely to show neurodevelop-mental delays of various types. Language milestones may be achieved later, and expressive language may be simple. Sensory motor coordination may be impaired, with poor handwriting and reading ability. These children are more likely to display behaviour problems at school, and there may be academic difficulties secondary to attention difficulties.

Oppositional and conduct disorders are very common and seem to be a complication of hyperactivity. Emotional disorders are also common and may be a result of failure at school and in interpersonal relationships.

Up to 10% of children with hyperactivity have autistic spectrum disorders, while nearly a third of children with autistic disorders meet the criteria for the diagnosis of ADHD (Santosh 2004). These children respond to treatment of hyperactivity. A number of children develop comorbid tic disorders in the early school years.

Some studies show high rates of overlap between ADHD and bipolar affective disorders. The relationship between ADHD and substance abuse is complex, with higher rates of ADHD in those seeking treatment for substance addiction. Children with ADHD who are followed up into early adulthood show increased rates of drug use and abuse. There is also some evidence that ADHD may act as an independent risk factor for substance abuse (Taylor *et al.* 2004).

Diagnosis and treatment

Diagnosis is made on clinical grounds using *DSM-IV* or *ICD-10* criteria. Screening tools such as the Connors rating scales for parents and teachers are useful for determining the child's behaviour profile in different situations. It is also helpful to see the child at school.

Anxiety and mood disorders, attachment disorders, conduct disorders without attention deficit and bipolar disorders should be considered in the differential diagnosis. Autistic disorders and learning disability may coexist with hyperkinetic disorders.

Psychological interventions, educational measures, medication and diet are all used for children with ADHD. Most children have many problems, and multi-mode intervention is usually necessary (*see* Chapter 8).

Other developmental disorders

These include specific disorders of speech and language, scholastic skills and motor function. The onset of symptoms is in infancy or childhood, and impairment or delay in development of functions is strongly related to biological maturation of the nervous system. Usually such impairment will diminish as the child gets older, although mild deficits often remain in adult life. These conditions are not diagnosed in children and adults with a learning disability, as their difficulties are part of their global impairment.

However, the disorder of motor coordination is often seen in children with ADHD and autism and may increase the disability of the child or adult. The concept of DAMP (deficits in attention, motor control and perception) has been in clinical use in Scandinavia for about 20 years, and is diagnosed on the basis of concomitant coordination disorder in children who do not have severe learning disability or cerebral palsy (Gillberg 2003).

Tic disorders

In children and adults with learning disability, tics are often seen in the context of autistic disorder and attention and hyperactivity disorders. In view of this association, it is useful to consider tic disorders here, although they are not developmental disorders.

A tic is an involuntary, rapid, recurrent, non-rhythmic, stereotyped motor movement or vocalisation that is of sudden onset and that serves no apparent purpose (*ICD-10*). Tics are common in school-age children and are usually transient. However, they can follow a more chronic course. The best known and studied of the tic disorders is Tourette's syndrome. The latter is defined by *ICD-10* as the presence of both multiple motor tics and one or more vocal tics over a period of more than 1 year during which there was not a tic-free period of more than 2 months, with an onset before 18 years. The definition in *DSM-IV-R* is similar. The other conditions include transient tic disorder, chronic motor tic disorder and chronic vocal tic disorder.

Tourette's syndrome

As defined above, Tourette's syndrome is a combined vocal and motor tic disorder with onset in childhood. Motor tics usually begin between the ages of 3 and 8 years with transient periods of eye blinking or some other facial tic (Leckman 2002). Vocal tics can begin as early as 3 years of age, but usually follow motor tics by several years. Simple motor tics are simple, sudden and meaningless muscle movements such as eye blinking, nose twitching or shoulder shrugging. Complex motor tics appear to be more purposeful and involve several muscle groups. Examples include touching other people or objects. Similarly, vocal tics can range from clearing the throat to utterance of words and sentences, including copro-lalia. Tic intensity can range from being barely noticeable to seriously interfering with everyday activities.

The tics show a waxing and waning course at different times of the day and over longer periods of time. Most patients have some control over their tics and describe premonitory urges preceding them which can be relieved by performing the tics.

Usually the onset of the tics is gradual, with mild tics alternating with tic-free periods. Facial tics are often the first to appear. In the following months and years the tics may spread to other parts of the body. Usually the tics peak in the second decade of life, with many affected individuals showing a striking reduction by the time they are 19 or 20 years of age. There appears to be an increased frequency of hyperactivity, impulsivity, attention impairment and obsessive-compulsive features in people with Tourette's syndrome.

A large epidemiological study (Khalifa and von Knorring 2003) reported that transient tics were present in up to 5% of school-age children, with a prevalence of Tourette's syndrome of 0.6%. Males are more often affected than females.

Neurobiology

There is convincing evidence that the basal ganglia and related cortico-striato-thalamo-cortical pathways are likely to be involved in both tics and related behavioural abnormalities (Hoekstra *et al.* 2004). It seems likely that specific neurotransmitter systems may be affected, particularly in view of the efficacy of dopamine-blocking medications in the treatment of tics.

Tourette's syndrome has a strong genetic background, but the phenotype may be variable and not confined to the full-blown syndrome. Family studies have shown that family members of the proband are more likely to have tics compared with the general population. At the present time no definite genetic locus has been identified.

A number of non-genetic factors have been implicated, particularly adverse perinatal events and infections. In recent years, post-infectious autoimmune mechanisms have also been considered in the pathogenesis of some cases of Tourette's syndrome. Tics have long been identified as stress-sensitive conditions, and there is often worsening of tics in relation to stressful life events, such as starting school.

Treatment

Treatment includes educational and supportive interventions in addition to medication. An informed and supportive home and school environment, good sleep hygiene and regular exercise can be beneficial (Leckman 2002). It is helpful if the interventions are provided in the context of a long-term relationship with a clinician who can help the patient. Psychotherapeutic interventions will help to address difficulties with self-esteem, social coping and family issues.

The drugs that are usually used in the treatment of Tourette's syndrome are dopamine-receptor-blocking drugs, both typical and atypical neuroleptics. It may also be necessary to treat concomitant inattention and hyperactivity. Serotonin reuptake inhibitors may also be needed in cases where there is comorbid obsessive-compulsive disorder.

Conclusion

Developmental disorders are often seen in children and adults with learning disability, and may colour the presentation of other conditions. They may also be mistaken for conditions such as schizophrenia. A person with an autistic disorder may be diagnosed as having treatment-resistant schizophrenia and may be treated accordingly, with poor results. A developmental perspective is invaluable if appropriate interventions are to be provided to enable the individual to achieve their full potential.

References

Acosta MT and Pearl PL (2003) The neurobiology of autism: new pieces of the puzzle. *Curr Neurol Neurosci Rep.* **3**: 149–56.

American Psychiatric Association (2000) *Diagnostic and Statistical Manual of Mental Disorders (4e). Text revision (DSM-IV-TR).* American Psychiatric Association, Washington, DC.

Baron-Cohen S (1997) *Mind Blindness: an essay on autism and theory of mind.* MIT Press, Cambridge, MA.

Baron-Cohen S (2003) *The Essential Difference: the truth about the male and female brain.* Basic Books, New York.

Biederman J and Faraone SV (2002) Current concepts in the neurobiology of attention deficit/hyperactivity disorder. *Attention Disord.* **6(Suppl. 1):** S7–16.

Blum K, Braverman ER, Holder JM *et al.* (2000). Reward deficiency syndrome: a biogenetic model for the diagnosis and treatment of impulsive, addictive and compulsive behaviors. *J Psychoactive Drugs.* **32(Suppl. i–iv):** 1–112.

Casanova MF, Buxhoeveden DP, Switala AE and Roy E (2002) Minicolumnar pathology in autism. *Neurology.* **58:** 428–32.

Duncan J (1986) Disorganization of behaviour after frontal lobe damage. *Cogn Neuropsychol.* **3:** 271–90.

Faraone SV and Biederman J (1994) Is attention deficit hyperactivity disorder familial? *Harvard Rev Psychiatry.* **1:** 271–87.

Fatemi SH, Stray JM, Halt AR and Realmuto GR (2001) Dysregulation of reelin and Bcl-2 proteins in autistic cerebellum. *J Autism Dev Disord.* **31:** 529–35.

Fombonne E (2003) Epidemiological surveys of autism and other pervasive developmental disorders: an update. *J Autism Dev Disord.* **33:** 365–82.

Frith C (2003) What do imaging studies tell us about the neural basis of autism? *Novartis Found Symp.* **251:** 149–66.

Gillberg C (2003) Deficits in attention, motor control and perception. *Arch Dis Child.* **88:** 904–10.

Hoekstra PJ, Anderson GM, Limburg PC, Korf J, Kallenberg CGM and Minderaa RB (2004) Neurobiology and neuroimmunology of Tourette's syndrome: an update. *Cell Mol Life Sci.* **61:** 886–98.

Humphrey N (1984) *Consciousness Regained. Chapters in the development of mind.* Oxford University Press, Oxford.

Kemper TL and Bauman M (1998) Neuropathology of infantile autism. *J Neuropathol Exp Neurol.* **57:** 645–52.

Khalifa N and von Knorring AL (2003) Prevalence of tic disorders and Tourette's syndrome in a Swedish school population. *Dev Med Child Neurol.* **45:** 315–19.

Leckman JF (2002) Tourette's syndrome. *Lancet.* **360:** 1577–86.

Lotter V (1966) Epidemiology of autistic conditions in young children. I. Prevalance. *J Am Soc Psych.* **1:** 124–37.

Nelson KB, Grether JK, Croen LA *et al.* (2001) Neuropeptides and neurotrophins in neonatal blood of children with autism or mental retardation. *Ann Neurol.* **49:** 597–606.

Ozonoff S, Cook I, Coon H *et al.* (2004) Performance on CANTAB subtests to frontal lobe function in people with autistic disorder: Evidence from the CPEA network. *J Autism Dev Disord.* **34:** 139–50.

Santosh P (2004) *Comorbidity of autism and ADHD. Paying attention to ADHD?* The Sixth International ADDISS Conference, Liverpool.

Sonuga-Barke EJS (2002) Psychological heterogeneity in ADHD: a dual-pathway model of behaviour and cognition. *Behav Brain Res.* **130:** 29–36.

Taylor E, Dopfner M, Sergeant J *et al.* (2004) European clinical guidelines for hyperkinetic disorder: first upgrade. *Eur Child Adolesc Psychiatry.* **13(Suppl. 1):** 7–30.

Thapar A, Holmes J, Poulton K and Harrington R (1999) Genetic basis of attention deficit and hyperactivity. *Br J Psychiatry.* **174:** 105–11.

Whitaker-Azmitia (2001) Serotonin and brain development: role in human development diseases. *Brain Res Bull.* **56(5):** 479–85.

Wing L (1996) *The Autistic Spectrum: a guide for parents and professionals.* Constable, London.

World Health Organization (1992) *ICD-10 Classification of Mental and Behavioural Disorders.* World Health Organization, Geneva.

Chapter 5

Epilepsy in people with intellectual disabilities

Geraldine Cassidy

Introduction

An epileptic seizure is a sudden paroxysmal, synchronous and repetitive discharge of cerebral neurons, the clinical manifestations of which depend on where the discharge started its spread and the duration of the discharge. Seizures result in interruptions to or abnormality in brain function, and may affect the level of consciousness, movement, sensation, and autonomic or psychic phenomena. They may be provoked but usually appear to be spontaneous. A person is said to have epilepsy if they have a recurrent tendency to experience seizures (Betts 1998).

Epileptiform activity starts at the cellular level and spreads to neighbouring cells which then discharge repeatedly and synchronously so that the epileptiform activity propagates and may involve other parts of the brain. It is mediated by neurotransmitters such as glutamate (which is excitatory) and gamma-amino-butyric acid (GABA) (which is inhibitory). Seizure activity may cause changes in the brain cells and even cell death.

Epilepsy and people with learning disabilities

Epilepsy is commonly associated with learning disability. People with learning disabilities and epilepsy deserve the best in epilepsy care, with the optimum balance being achieved between seizure control and minimisation of adverse effects from treatment. For the affected individual, epilepsy entails more than seizures and their quality of life will depend on non-medical aspects of management, such as carer attitudes to epilepsy and to the taking of calculated risks.

Total population surveys on prevalence suggest that 5 to 10 in 1000 people suffer from epilepsy (defined as two or more seizures, at least one of which occurred in the previous five years and/or receiving drug treatment for epilepsy). The prevalence of epilepsy increases in patients with concurrent neurological disorders and also depends on the severity of learning disability. Earlier studies of epilepsy in people with learning disabilities show various methodological errors, such as the use of non-standardised definitions and institutionalised study samples. These factors overestimate the prevalence of epilepsy. Prevalence rates in adults with mild, moderate, severe and profound learning disability have been reported to be 4%, 7%, 12% and 28%, respectively (Lund 1985). This chapter will address the complex interaction between epilepsy and learning disabilities, causation, assessment and treatment, and the role of staff within learning

51

disability services. In addition, the relationship between epilepsy, mental illness and behaviour disorders will be explored.

Causes of epilepsy and classification

In many cases, the aetiology or cause of the learning disability and that of the epilepsy are the same, each disability being the consequence of brain damage arising either before or after birth. In the classification system of the Commission on Classification and Terminology of the International League Against Epilepsy (ILAE) (1989), individuals with a known cause of their epilepsy who have significant brain abnormality are said to have symptomatic epilepsy. The term *cryptogenic epilepsy* is used when no significant brain abnormality is found but it is presumed to be symptomatic. In individuals for whom the causation is unknown, the term *idiopathic epilepsy* is used. Many cases of epilepsy in people with learning disabilities are therefore symptomatic.

Causes can be categorised as genetic or acquired. Genetic causes include chromosomal abnormalities (e.g. Down syndrome or fragile X syndrome) and single gene defects (e.g. tuberous sclerosis, phenylketonuria). Acquired disorders include infections such as meningitis and encephalitis, metabolic disorders, brain tumours, trauma or haemorrhage. Premature infants are particularly vulnerable to metabolic disorders and brain haemorrhage in the perinatal period. People with Down syndrome may have epileptic seizures with ageing in association with the onset of Alzheimer-type dementia, in which case the outcome is poor.

Given the wide variety of disorders that may be associated with both epilepsy and learning disability, it is important that individuals presenting with seizures are assessed carefully to find the underlying cause. The neurocutaneous disorders, which affect the nervous system and skin (e.g. tuberous sclerosis, neurofibromatosis and Sturge–Weber's syndrome), are particularly important due to the likely involvement of several body systems and the need for genetic counselling for family members. With a full knowledge of the underlying causation it is easier to give information on the prognosis and to select appropriate therapy.

In 1981, the Commission on Classification and Terminology of the International League Against Epilepsy (ILAE) proposed the classification of seizures on the basis of whether both hemispheres of the brain were affected, and the level of consciousness. Partial seizures originate from one cerebral hemisphere. When consciousness is not impaired it is classified as a simple partial seizure. When consciousness is impaired, it is classified as a complex partial seizure. In generalised seizures, the first clinical changes indicate initial involvement of both hemispheres. Consciousness may be impaired, and this may be the initial manifestation. Epileptic activity in partial seizures may spread to the other hemisphere, and this is called secondary generalisation. A person with learning disabilities may be unable to give a clear account of their seizures, and it is likely that partial seizures are often missed in this population. They may have multiple seizures or seizures that are difficult to classify. Videotelemetry electroencephalogram (EEG) or ambulatory EEG recording may be useful in such instances where there is marked diagnostic uncertainty.

Epilepsy can also be classified according to syndromes (Commission on Classification and Terminology of the International League Against Epilepsy 1989). The ILAE recognises a number of epilepsy syndromes, which are determined by age of onset, seizure type, EEG abnormality and associated neurological abnormality. Epileptic syndromes with an onset early in life are associated with a poorer outcome. West's syndrome and Lennox–Gastaut's syndrome are of particular importance, as they are manifested in childhood and may lead to significant learning disabilities. Seizures in the newborn suggest a brain insult arising around the time of birth. Both morbidity and mortality are high, and many of these cases go on to develop epilepsy or learning disability.

In West's syndrome, there is a characteristic EEG appearance of hypsarrhythmia (a chaotic mixture of high-amplitude slow waves with variable spike and sharp waves) and infantile spasms, with most affected children going on to have severe learning disabilities and chronic epilepsy. Seizures typically start between 6 and 9 months of age and show a limited response to treatment, although some success has been achieved with benzodiazepines, adrenocorticotropic hormone (ACTH) and vigabatrin. Lennox–Gastaut's syndrome presents with intractable seizures, which are mixed in type and are associated with learning disability. Again there is a characteristic EEG appearance (diffuse, slow spike and waves between seizures, and bursts of fast activity in sleep). This disorder has its onset in the 2 to 6 years age group and may follow on from West's syndrome. Over 90% of affected children have learning disabilities in the long term.

Sufficient information may not be available to make precise distinction between symptomatic, idiopathic and cryptogenic epilepsy, particularly for adults with learning disabilities. For example, Mariani *et al.* (1993) could classify only 28% of cases into specific syndromes. However, for the great majority of cases, classification into partial or generalised seizure types is possible, and is crucial to ensure selection of the correct anti-epileptic medication.

Classification of seizures

Seizures are classified as generalised or partial. The full classification is presented in Box 5.1.

Box 5.1 Classification of seizures

Simple partial seizures (without impairment of consciousness)
With motor signs
With somatosensory or special sensory symptoms
With autonomic symptoms
With psychic symptoms

Complex partial seizures (with impairment of consciousness)
Beginning as simple partial and progressing to impairment of consciousness
With impairment of consciousness from onset

Partial seizure evolving into secondarily generalised seizure
Generalised seizures
Typical absence
Atypical absence
Myoclonic seizures
Clonic seizures

Tonic seizures
Tonic–clonic seizures
Atonic seizures
Unclassified seizures
Information for classification inadequate or incomplete

Clinical descriptions

Generalised seizures

Tonic–clonic seizures (grand mal in previous classifications)

This primary generalised seizure starts without any warning. There is a sudden cry followed by total muscular rigidity, falling and powerful jerking movements of all four limbs, usually lasting for less than 2 minutes. This is followed by a phase of unresponsive coma lasting for a few minutes. There may be seizure-related injuries and emptying of the bladder, and the person may remain confused for up to 24 hours.

Absence seizures

Typically absence (or petit mal) seizures occur in children and are characterised by three-per-minute spike and slow waves in the EEG. The child may have a brief lapse of consciousness lasting for less than 45 seconds, during which time eye blinking, myoclonus or drop attacks may be observed. Typical absences are rare in adults of normal intelligence, but are seen in adults with learning disabilities. Atypical absences may appear to be clinically similar, but the EEG appearance is quite different. They are usually found with other forms of epilepsy.

Myoclonic seizures

There is stereotyped jerking of all or some of the limbs with or without jerking of the head. Myoclonic seizures are more often seen in people with learning disabilities in conjunction with other forms of epilepsy, and may be difficult to control.

Atonic seizures

There is a sudden loss of postural tone associated with a fall. There is a risk of significant injury with these seizures.

Partial seizures

Simple partial seizures

There is no disturbance of consciousness in these seizures. If the motor cortex is involved, as in the commonest form of simple partial seizures, there may be focal spasms of a group of muscles. This kind of epilepsy has been termed Jacksonian epilepsy. There may a period of paralysis in the affected muscles, known as Todd's paralysis. Sensory seizures are rarer. There may be a sensation of pins and needles. Visual and auditory hallucinations and auras of taste and smell are other examples of simple sensory seizures.

Complex partial seizures

In complex partial seizures there is disturbance of consciousness. Automatisms occur, ranging from simple ones such as chewing and smacking of the lips to complex semi-purposive behaviours such as undressing and walking. The seizure usually lasts for less than 5 minutes, but complex partial status epilepticus (in which the epileptic activity goes on for a prolonged period of time) may occur, particularly in people with learning disabilities. The individual can present with a wide variety of symptoms, such as irritability, wandering and psychosis. All partial seizures, both simple and complex, can evolve into generalised seizures.

Status epilepticus

This refers to a continuous succession of seizures occurring without any period of recovery. Both generalised and partial seizures can produce status epilepticus. Generalised convulsive status epilepticus is defined as two or more seizures without full recovery or more or less continuous seizure activity for 30 minutes or more. This is a medical emergency due to the potential for profound neuronal and systemic damage. It can occur if anti-epileptic medication is withdrawn abruptly or is taken irregularly.

Assessment

The diagnosis of epilepsy is essentially a clinical one based on an accurate eyewitness description of seizures. Patients with learning disabilities are usually unable to describe the complex and often unpleasant pre-ictal or ictal experiences. The doctor who is making the assessment needs to consider other disorders which may be mistaken for epilepsy, including faints, cardiac arrhythmias, transient ischaemic attacks, non-epileptic seizures and behavioural disorders. Information on the seizures themselves should include a description of the person before, during and after the event, noting any precipitants such as anxiety or infection. Some medications, particularly antidepressants and antipsychotics, increase the likelihood of seizures in susceptible individuals, and in such cases withdrawal of the offending drug may be all that is required. A developmental history should be taken, followed by an assessment of skills and disabilities. Information on behaviour and personality should be obtained because of the relationship between seizures and behavioural disorders. Mental state and cognitive examinations are also important, together with an assessment of associated psychiatric disorder and the degree of cognitive impairment.

Patients who are attending an epilepsy clinic for the first time will usually undergo a physical examination to assess their general physical and nutritional status, the side-effects of any medication and seizure-related injuries. Physical stigmata of disorders that are known to cause learning disability and epilepsy should be noted.

Investigations will include baseline haematological and biochemical profiles. Screening for metabolic and degenerative disorders is usual, particularly in children presenting with learning disability and epilepsy. In the past, measurement of anti-epileptic serum levels has been performed excessively, and this should not be considered a routine part of monitoring. It may be appropriate after commencement of anti-epileptic medication, if there is suspicion of toxicity, or if there is failure to control seizures and it is thought that a low dose or non-compliance with medication may be responsible for this.

A baseline electroencephalogram (EEG) examination will form part of the initial assessment. This test records brain electrical activity by means of electrodes placed on the head. The EEG must be interpreted with caution, as a proportion of people with epilepsy have normal recordings between seizures, and some show epileptiform abnormalities in the absence of clinical symptoms. It may be difficult to achieve a satisfactory recording in some people with learning disabilities who may be frightened by the procedure, and the role of familiar staff in providing support and reassurance in such situations cannot be overestimated. Some EEG providers offer a domiciliary service whereby the technicians go into homes, schools and day services, which may be more acceptable to patients with learning disabilities. In some cases sedation may be required. The use of the unlicensed medication melatonin as pre-medication to induce sleep will increase the likelihood of epileptiform activity being seen without altering the EEG sleep architecture. Ambulatory recordings and video telemetry are useful for elucidating the relationship between seizures and behaviour, or when non-epileptic seizures are suspected.

Various forms of neuroimaging, including computerised tomography (CT), magnetic resonance imaging (MRI), single photon emission computerised tomography (SPECT) and positron emission tomography (PET) are useful for identifying focal lesions, particularly as a part of pre-surgical assessment. MRI is the investigation of choice in epilepsy. Sedation or even a general anaesthetic may be necessary if neuroimaging is to be completed in patients with severe learning disabilities. If surgical treatment is being considered, a referral to a specialist centre for neuropsychological tests and full work-up will be needed.

Management

The management of epilepsy in people with learning disabilities requires the co-operative and collaborative working of the multi-disciplinary team. The person who has been given the diagnosis will often receive input from several agencies. These may include staff from the primary healthcare team, school, day services, respite care, specialist nurses, physiotherapy, speech therapy and clinical psychology, as well as doctors specialising in epilepsy or learning disability psychiatry.

The diagnosis of epilepsy may come as a considerable shock to carers and may result in a grief reaction. Information on the condition may need to be repeated, as carers may not be able to absorb the information given at the first appointment. Carer education and support represent an essential element of epilepsy management and can be provided by specialist nurses, such as community learning disability nurses. Carers value information on the treatment and prognosis of epilepsy.

Drug therapy

Anti-epileptic drugs, their indications for use and common side-effects are listed in Table 5.1.

Table 5.1 Anti-epileptic drugs

Anti-epileptic drug	Indications for use	Side-effects
Sodium valproate	Broad spectrum of activity, suitable for all seizure types	Gastric irritation, tremor, weight gain, hair loss
Carbamazepine	Partial and generalised seizures, except absences	Nausea and vomiting, sedation, double vision, leukopenia, dizziness, headache
Lamotrigine	Suitable for all seizure types	Skin rashes, ataxia, double vision, Stevens–Johnson syndrome
Clonazepam	Suitable for all seizure types	Sedation
Clobazam	Suitable for all seizure types	Sedation
Vigabatrin	Partial and secondarily generalised seizures, West's syndrome	Drowsiness, dizziness, adverse behavioural effects, psychosis, visual field defects
Gabapentin	Add-on therapy in partial seizures	Somnolence, dizziness, ataxia
Ethosuximide	Absence seizures only	Nausea, anorexia, vomiting
Phenobarbitone	All forms of epilepsy except absence seizures	Fatigue, listlessness, depression, insomnia, behavioural disturbance
Phenytoin	All forms of epilepsy except absence seizures	Ataxia, nausea, sedation, gingival hyperplasia
Levetiracetam	Add-on therapy for partial seizures	Somnolence, dizziness, headache
Topiramate	Add-on therapy for partial seizures	Cognitive slowing, speech disorders, renal stones, weight loss
Tiagabine	Add-on therapy for partial seizures	Sedation, dizziness, ataxia, rash
Oxcarbazepine	Monotherapy or add-on therapy for partial seizures with or without generalised tonic–clonic seizures	Fatigue, dizziness, headache, somnolence, nausea, vomiting, rash

The majority of people with epilepsy will require the prescription of anti-epileptic medication. In some cases, particularly where there is severe brain damage, it may not be possible to completely eliminate seizures without causing excessive side-effects such as sedation or cognitive impairment, and the prescribing doctor must balance the risks and benefits involved. Selection of the anti-epileptic drugs will depend on the type of seizure, the syndromic classification (if known) and individual patient factors.

The vast majority of people can be treated with one or two drugs. Polytherapy should be avoided, due to the likelihood of increased side-effects which the patient may be unable to report. The dose should be increased gradually, noting any adverse side-effects. Carbamazepine and sodium valproate remain the drugs most widely used for this purpose in the UK. Newer drugs are being used more frequently either in monotherapy (lamotrigine) or as an adjunct (gabapentin, topiramate, levetiracetam), and this trend is supported by recent guidance from the National Institute for Clinical Excellence (2004). Older drugs such as phenytoin and phenobarbitone are no longer the treatment of first choice, due to the potential for side-effects.

The benzodiazepines clobazam and clonazepam are used as add-on therapies, their usefulness being limited by the development of tolerance. One exception is the use of clobazam as a prophylactic treatment for women who experience a cluster of seizures in the premenstrual phase. Once started on drug therapy, it is important that seizures are recorded accurately. This can be a problem, particularly when the person spends time in several settings, and the use of a seizure diary is essential.

Diazepam is administered rectally to patients who experience prolonged or serial seizures. It is absorbed rapidly and has anticonvulsant, anxiolytic, sedative and muscle-relaxant effects. It can be administered in family homes, day services, etc. by carers or staff who have received training. Written protocols or guidelines for use of rectal diazepam should be available, and should document when to give this treatment, the dosage, when to call for assistance, etc. An alternative rescue medication is midazolam, a benzodiazepine drug commonly used in anaesthesia which, although unlicensed for the purpose, is being used with positive effects via the buccal route (which is preferred by users and carers alike). In the general population, the majority of people will have their seizures adequately controlled using drug therapy and may not need specialist follow-up. However, people with a learning disability may continue to have intractable seizures and require ongoing specialist support. Primary healthcare teams may have limited experience of working with this client group, and general neurology services may not adequately meet their needs either. The learning disability team is therefore well placed to provide treatment and follow-up, given their expertise in the field.

Non-drug treatments

Surgical treatments should be considered in cases where seizures are resistant to drug therapy and where a resectable lesion is believed to be the focus of epileptic activity. Pre-surgical evaluation will be needed to document the precise location of the lesion and to weigh up the risks and benefits of surgery. Vagal nerve stimulation (VNS) may offer hope to patients with pharmacoresistant epilepsy. VNS therapy uses a small device inserted into the chest which stimulates the left vagal nerve, thus reducing seizures. People with learning disabilities have been helped by surgery, and referral for surgical evaluation should be considered as part of management.

Specific diets, including the ketogenic diet, have been used in the management of seizures that prove unresponsive to drug therapy, particularly in children. The diet is rather unpalatable, and parents will require support from a dietitian to comply with the requirements exactly.

Non-pharmacological approaches to seizure control can be divided into measures aimed at reducing seizure frequency and those that focus on improving psychological adjustment to epilepsy. In reflex epilepsy where specific triggers for seizures exist, the person can be advised to avoid these triggers (e.g. flickering lights). Many people report an increase in seizures in association with anxiety, and a variety of relaxation strategies have been used to reduce anxiety symptoms. The use of alternative therapies such as aromatherapy and reflexology has also been reported. Lifestyle-focused approaches, including advice on exercise, have been found to reduce seizure frequency.

Living with epilepsy

To avoid overprotection and an overly restricted lifestyle, carers and people with epilepsy need advice and education, including the following:

1 information on epilepsy, including aetiology, seizure types, prognosis, recording of seizures, etc.
2 anti-epileptic medication, side-effects, compliance, missed doses, etc.
3 seizure triggers
4 effects on lifestyle (i.e. safety at home and at work, sports, etc.)
5 first aid for seizures, including the management of status epilepticus
6 sources of information and support (e.g. voluntary agencies, specialist nurses).

People with epilepsy face some legal restrictions, notably in the areas of driving and employment. Research in mainstream epilepsy has focused on the quality of life of the person with epilepsy, and on stress and adjustment in carers.

The use of outcome measures to assess response to treatment may be helpful. Seizures diaries provide information on seizure frequency and duration and the use of rescue medication. It can be difficult to assess the effect of seizures on quality of life in a person who is already disabled, and further research is needed in this area, although a number of scales have been developed for this purpose, such as the Epilepsy Outcome Scale (Espie *et al.* 1998).

Behavioural and psychiatric disorders

Until the last century, epilepsy was considered to be a mental disorder and those affected by the condition were often residents in psychiatric institutions. Epilepsy is now accepted as a neurological disorder and it is known that not all people with epilepsy (or epilepsy and learning disability) have a psychiatric disorder. Psychiatric symptoms occur in the prodromal phase that occurs hours (or rarely days) before a seizure, during seizures (particularly those that are simple or complex partial in type) and postictally (when confusion, aggression and dysthymic mood may be present). These symptoms are most likely to respond to adjustments in anti-epileptic drug treatment, which improves seizure control.

Interictal psychiatric symptoms or disorders may be short-lived or lengthy in duration. The aetiology is multifactorial, reflecting the interaction of personality, family relationships, and societal responses to epilepsy and disability in addition to the epilepsy and its treatment. Rates of affective (mood) disorders and suicide are raised in people with normal intelligence and epilepsy, and a link to right-hemispheric EEG abnormality has been suggested. The diagnosis of psychiatric disorder is difficult in people with learning disabilities, particularly in those with a severe learning disability. Deb and Hunter (1991) did not find increased rates of affective disorder when they compared adults with learning disability with and without epilepsy. Psychosis and depression have been seen in those taking vigabatrin (which in someone with a learning disability may present with a behaviour disorder), and have also been described with other anti-epileptics.

Cognitive deterioration may be seen in chronic epilepsy, and may be due to repetitive seizure-related head injuries and/or episodes of status epilepticus.

Behaviour disorders are common in people with learning disabilities, and are multifactorial in aetiology. Carers are often most distressed by behavioural problems that can result in diminution in quality of life due to a reduction in access to community facilities and services. In their study, Deb and Hunter (1991) found a subgroup of people with epilepsy, mild learning disabilities and generalised EEG abnormality who had more challenging behaviours. A change of anti-epileptic medication can result in deterioration in behaviour despite improved seizure control. This may be short-lived, but if severe it may prove unacceptable to carers. Behaviour disorders may be unrelated to the epilepsy and its treatment. After easily treated medical conditions such as ear infections have been ruled out, a careful functional analysis based on detailed descriptions of behaviour and/or observation by a professional skilled in working with people with learning disabilities is necessary to achieve an understanding of the behaviour and to provide advice on management.

Concluding remarks

Epilepsy is a common additional disability in people with learning disabilities, with seizures continuing into adulthood and in a substantial proportion of cases proving resistant to anti-epileptic drug therapy. The accurate diagnosis of epilepsy is dependent on a good account of seizures from carers, who also have an important role in management. The selection of drug therapy should be based on a classification of seizures and/or epileptic syndrome according to international guidelines, and must balance the risks and benefits. Management should address the social and psychological aspects as well as the purely medical ones. Behavioural and psychiatric disorders are not always present in people with epilepsy and learning disabilities, but when present merit a careful assessment to find the underlying causes.

References

Betts T (1998) *Epilepsy, Psychiatry and Learning Difficulty.* Martin Dunitz, London.

Commission on Classification and Terminology of the International League Against Epilepsy (1981) Proposal for revised clinical and electroencephalographic classification of epileptic seizures. *Epilepsia.* **22:** 489–501.

Commission on Classification and Terminology of the International League Against Epilepsy (1989) Proposal for revised classification of epilepsies and epileptic syndromes. *Epilepsia.* **30:** 389–99.

Deb S and Hunter D (1991) Psychopathology of people with mental handicap and epilepsy I–III. *Br J Psychiatry.* **59:** 822–34.

Espie C, Paul A, Graham M *et al.* (1998) The Epilepsy Outcome Scale: the development of a measure for use with carers of people with epilepsy plus intellectual disability. *J Intellect Disabil Res.* **42:** 90–96.

Lund J (1985) Epilepsy and psychiatric disorder in the mentally retarded adult. *Acta Psychiatr Scand.* **72:** 557–62.

Mariani E, Ferini-Strambi L, Sala M *et al.* (1993) Epilepsy in institutionalised patients with encephalopathy: clinical aspects and nosological considerations. *Am J Ment Retard.* **98(Suppl.):** 27–33.

National Institute for Clinical Excellence (2004) *Newer Drugs for Epilepsy in Adults. Technology Appraisal 76;* www.nice.org.uk.

Chapter 6

Common syndromes and genetic disorders

David Clarke

Introduction and terminology

This chapter provides an introduction to the concept of syndromes and describes some genetically determined syndromes that are or may be associated with learning disability. Some basic genetic terms and concepts are discussed in Chapter 2. Terms that are used to describe how common diseases are include incidence and prevalence. The incidence of a disease is the rate of occurrence of new cases in a defined population over a given period of time. Prevalence is the proportion of a defined population that has a disease at a given point in time or over a given period of time.

Syndromes

A syndrome is a characteristic pattern of clinical features. Such features include signs that a clinician can see or otherwise ascertain, such as a rash or heart murmur, and symptoms which a patient may experience, such as pain or low mood. This chapter deals with syndromes that cause or may cause learning disability. Such disorders include Down syndrome and fragile X syndrome, both of which are relatively common. People with learning disability may have other syndromes, such as Beçet's syndrome (a combination of oral and genital ulceration, believed to result from immunological abnormalities). Such syndromes are coincidental or secondary rather than causal.

There can be disadvantages to the 'labelling' of people with disabilities, but the diagnosis of a syndrome has many benefits for the person concerned and their carers. These include an explanation of the cause of the person's disabilities or of their pattern of strengths and weaknesses, improved knowledge regarding the risk of recurrence of the disorder among relatives if a syndrome is of genetic origin, and the prediction of other features that may not be apparent to the person concerned or their carers, but which may be medically or educationally important. Such features might include the likelihood of heart disease, or of a discrepancy between verbal and non-verbal cognitive ability. People who have syndromes associated with heart defects may need antibiotic cover for some types of dental work or other invasive surgery.

Other advantages include the prediction of features that may develop in the future. This is particularly important when treatment can alleviate the problem (e.g. the disorders of thyroid function to which people with Down syndrome are susceptible). It may also be important in allowing relatives to plan for the future (e.g. through knowledge of the increased risk of dementia of Alzheimer type associated with Down syndrome).

Diagnosis also provides access to support groups. People with syndromes and their carers may increase their knowledge and their ability to access services through membership of such a group. Parents and carers often feel less isolated when they know that other people face similar problems, and they may find practical solutions to their difficulties of which professionals are not aware. An alphabetical list of support organisations is given in the *Contact a Family (CaF) Directory* (www.cafamily.org.uk).

Behavioural phenotypes

Behavioural and cognitive aspects are so striking and characteristic a feature of some syndromes that they may be used to prompt diagnostic assessment. Examples include the severe self-injury associated with Lesch–Nyhan syndrome, and the combination of appetite abnormality, ritualistic behaviours, sleep abnormalities, skin picking, repetitive speech and vulnerability to psychiatric disorder associated with Prader–Willi syndrome. Such patterns of vulnerability to particular emotional or behavioural problems or peculiarities associated with biologically determined syndromes have been termed behavioural phenotypes. Environmental factors may interact with vulnerability to a particular behaviour to determine whether or not it occurs in a given setting, and this interaction may be important for determining effective treatments. For example, in Lesch–Nyhan disease all affected men self-injure, but whether a man with the syndrome injures himself at a particular time is influenced by environmental and internal psychological factors such as stress and anxiety.

Syndrome descriptions

Down syndrome

J Langdon Down originally described this disorder in 1887. Trisomy 21 was first reported in association with Down syndrome in 1958. About 1 in 600 liveborn children have Down syndrome. The rate increases with increasing maternal age, being about 1 in 1400 at a maternal age of 25 years and 1 in 30 at a maternal age of 45 years. There are three types of abnormalities affecting chromosome 21. In about 95% of cases Down syndrome is caused by primary non-disjunction (failure of separation of chromosomes during egg or sperm production) leading to trisomy 21. The risk of recurrence of this abnormality is low if maternal age is also relatively low. In about 2% of cases Down syndrome results from an unbalanced translocation when material from one chromosome breaks off and 'sticks' to another. This often involves chromosomes 21 and 14, and is usually a 'one-off' event. In some cases a parent also has a balanced translocation with no overall disruption or duplication of genetic material, and here the risk of recurrence is high. Chromosome 21 to chromosome 21 translocations can also occur. Mosaicism is a term used to describe the presence of two or more cell lines within the body. In Down syndrome, this means that there may be one cell line with trisomy 21 and one unaffected cell line. In about 3% of cases the syndrome probably results from mosaicism. Many cases may not be diagnosed. The proportion of affected and unaffected cell lines varies, as does the degree of intellectual impairment.

There is usually 'floppiness' or muscular hypotonia at birth which usually improves with development. Most adults are of short stature, with a characteristic facial appearance. The eyes seem to slope upwards and outwards as a result of alterations in the structure of the surrounding tissues. The nose has a wide bridge, and the head has an unusual shape, being broader than long (brachycephaly). Limb abnormalities include a single transverse crease on the palm, a large cleft between the first and second toes, and relatively short upper arms. People with Down syndrome are prone to abnormalities of the thyroid gland, with 15% developing hypothyroidism during childhood or adolescence. About 50% have a heart abnormality. Abnormalities of the gastrointestinal tract occur in a significant minority of cases. Life expectancy has improved markedly over the past 50 years, largely as a result of antibiotic treatment of respiratory tract infections. Survival into the eighth decade is unusual but not extraordinary. The presence of a serious heart defect may lead to heart and lung failure in early adult life. Adults with Down syndrome are much more likely to develop dementia of Alzheimer type than the general population. On post-mortem examination, almost all adults with Down syndrome over the age of 35 years have the brain changes characteristic of dementia of Alzheimer type. However, only about 45% of those over 45 years of age have clinically apparent dementia. Changes in blood cells are relatively common. Older texts reported an association between Down syndrome and leukaemia, but recent research suggests that leukaemia is rare, affecting less than 1% of people with Down syndrome.

The stereotypical image of people with Down syndrome as happy, placid individuals with a gift for mimicry is not borne out by recent behavioural research. Stubbornness and obsessional features seem to be over-represented, and many people with Down syndrome react adversely in situations involving changes to expected routines or conflict. Autism occurs more commonly than would be expected by chance alone.

Most adults with Down syndrome have a moderate learning disability. About 10% have low-normal intelligence (i.e. cognitive impairments that are not so severe as to be classifiable as a learning disability). Almost all children with Down syndrome have some degree of specific speech and language delay. About 25% have features of attention deficit disorder. Cognitive abilities tend to be greater among people whose Down syndrome is caused by mosaicism for trisomy 21. Further information may be obtained at www.downs-syndrome.org.uk.

Fragile X syndrome

All ethnic groups are affected equally, with a frequency of about 0.3–1 per 1000 in men and 0.2–0.6 per 1000 in women. Fragile X syndrome is an X-linked disorder, but has a very unusual pattern of inheritance. X-linked disorders such as haemophilia are usually manifested in men who have one X chromosome, and are transmitted by unaffected women carriers who have two X chromosomes. Fragile X syndrome is characterised by a bias towards affected men, but with some affected women and some unaffected men who transmit the abnormality to their daughters, who then have affected sons. When peripheral blood lymphocytes from affected individuals are grown in certain culture conditions, including a lack of folic acid, a fragile site becomes evident on the long (q) arm of the X chromosome at Xq27.3 (fragile site A). Fragile sites may not be seen in some unaffected men who transmit the abnormality to their carrier daughters. These men are termed 'normal transmitting males'. The probability that a child with a fragile X chromosome will have learning disability depends on the sex and intellect of the parent from whom the chromosome was inherited.

The 'fragility' of the X chromosome is now known to be associated with an unstable region of DNA within the fragile X mental retardation (FMR-1) gene. This region of unstable DNA gradually increases in length and degree of instability in successive generations (a pre-mutation) until a critical point is reached and the gene no longer functions (a full mutation). The instability is caused by an increase in CGG (cytosine–guanine–guanine) repeats from the 50 or so repeats that are usual to 50–100 repeats (pre-mutation) to over 200 repeats (full mutation). The likelihood of a child inheriting a lengthened gene is proportional to the length of the unstable region in the carrier mother. An increase does not occur in the children of normal transmitting males. Modern genetic testing for fragile X syndrome involves analysing the relevant portion of DNA for CGG repeats (rather than looking for fragile sites). The severity of intellectual disability and other fragile-X-related phenomena in women probably depends on the proportion of cells in which the abnormal chromosome is inactivated as they 'use' one copy of their two X chromosomes, inactivation being random. Variants of fragile X syndrome (FraX-A) have now been identified, with DNA expansions nearer to the tip of the X chromosome's long arm. These include FraX-E and FraX-F.

The physical features of this syndrome are variable. The most characteristic feature is that about 95% of affected men have large testes. Unfortunately, this is not usually apparent until after puberty (thus precluding the use of this finding to aid early diagnosis). Other features include a long face with a large forehead, large simple ears, a large lower jaw and a high-arched palate. There is a connective tissue disorder which may lead to tissue laxity, hyper-extensible joints, flat feet, heart defects (especially valve abnormalities) and ear infections (because the Eustachian tube connecting the ear to the respiratory tract closes easily). Eye abnormalities such as cataracts may occur and lead to impaired vision. About 50% of affected men have epilepsy. Life expectancy depends on the severity of associated features such as epilepsy and heart problems, but is probably nearly normal.

There is usually some degree of social impairment, with social anxiety and avoidance of eye-to-eye contact, but with social responsiveness. Men with fragile X syndrome are usually affectionate, and do not have the aloof quality typical of autism. Self-injury is relatively common, especially hand biting over the anatomical snuff-box (between the thumb and index finger) in response to frustration, anxiety or excitement. Stereotyped behaviours such as hand flapping are not uncommon.

The learning disability is usually mild to moderate. Verbal intelligence scores exceed performance scores among populations of affected men and non-disabled women carriers. Some studies have found that the rate of intellectual development diminishes with age after puberty. Simultaneous information-processing abilities are greater than sequential processing skills. Speech and language development is delayed, with dysfluent conversation, incomplete sentences, echolalia and verbal perseveration (an inability to move on from the subject being discussed). Speech is often disorganised, with poor topic maintenance and tangential comments. It may be rapid, or include peculiar changes in pitch. There may be problems with attention and concentration that are disproportionate to the severity of the associated learning disability. Hyperactivity may be the presenting feature among boys with fragile X syndrome who do not have a learning disability. Further information can be obtained at www.fragilex.org.uk.

Alpha mannosidosis

Alpha mannosidosis is one of a family of lysosomal storage disorders. It is inherited by autosomal recessive transmission, and the gene has been mapped to chromosome 19. Clinical features include a characteristic facial appearance, with a prominent forehead, a flattened nasal bridge, a small nose and a broad mouth. There are usually signs of cerebellar dysfunction with abnormal gait. A hearing impairment is caused by nerve dysfunction as well as an accumulation of fluid in the middle ear leading to a reduction in sound transfer. Language abnormalities include delayed speech development with incomplete sentences, restricted vocabulary and a lack of understanding of abstract concepts. There is an immunological deficiency caused by reduced immunoglobulin response to infections, and a reduction in the ability of white blood cells to destroy infectious agents. Bone, joint and muscle abnormalities may occur, with accumulation of storage material in muscle tissue.

Unpublished information suggests an association with severe psychiatric disorder with affective and psychotic symptoms, often including some features similar to an organic confusional state, and with excessive sleepiness towards the end of episodes. Further information may be found at www.mannosidosis.org.

Angelman syndrome

The prevalence of this syndrome is estimated at 1 in 30 000 births. Most cases are sporadic, and are associated with deletions within 15q11q13 of maternal origin (cf. Prader–Willi syndrome). Angelman syndrome is occasionally associated with paternal uniparental disomy (i.e. both the chromosome 15s are of paternal origin, so that the maternal chromosome 15 has been 'deleted'), but this seems to be less common than in Prader–Willi syndrome. A gene responsible for the Angelman syndrome phenotype has recently been described (Koshino *et al.* 1997).

Physical characteristics include a small head, a characteristic face with a wide mouth, a 'hooked' nose, a prominent lower jaw, widely spaced teeth and tongue protrusion. Many affected children are hypopigmented compared with first-degree relatives. Voluntary movements are jerky and the gait is ataxic with stiff legs. About 80% of cases develop epilepsy, and the EEG is highly characteristic. There are no data available at the present time about life expectancy, but it is likely that this is potentially normal.

Behavioural characteristics, which include sudden bursts of laughter, together with the physical features led to the term 'happy puppet' syndrome being employed in the 1960s and 1970s. These children enjoy social and physical contact, and mouthing objects. Many are fascinated by water. They have severe learning disabilities and delayed motor milestones. There is little speech development (no reported cases have more than six words), but their understanding of language may be better. Overactivity is often associated with a short attention span. Further information can be obtained at www.assert.dial.pipex.com/.

Apert's syndrome

E Apert described this syndrome in 1906. The prevalence is approximately 1 per 180 000 liveborn infants. It is an autosomal dominant condition, but most cases arise as new mutations (i.e. with unaffected parents). Recent research has demonstrated a point mutation in a gene on chromosome 10 (fibroblast growth factor receptor 2 or FGFR2) (Britto *et al.* 2001)

   Physical features include a high, prominent forehead, often with midline swelling, a small flattened nose, under-development of the middle portion of the face and abnormalities of the oral cavity and lower jaw leading to feeding, breathing or speech problems, shallow eye sockets and large prominent eyes set widely apart, low set ears, often with conductive hearing impairment, and hydrocephalus in some cases. Many of the abnormalities result from premature fusion of the 'plates' that contribute to skull development. Hand malformations include syndactyly (fusion of the second/third/fourth fingers) and 'claw-like' fingers. Skin disorders include severe acne during adolescence. Heart and kidney abnormalities may also occur. Life expectancy depends on the severity of the clinical features and associated complications and is potentially normal. Hyper-activity is reported to be over-represented. IQ ranges from normal to moderate learning disability. Social problems and lack of confidence may result from facial disabilities. Articulation problems are common but are usually due to facial abnormalities rather than central mechanisms. Clinicians should be alert to the possible presence of sleep apnoea syndrome. Further information can be obtained at www.apert.org.

Coffin–Lowry syndrome

The incidence and prevalence of this syndrome are unknown, but more than 100 cases have been reported. This X-linked syndrome has been ascribed to a locus in the Xp22.1-p22.2 region. Physical features include short stature, coarse facial appearance with slanting eye fissures, a prominent forehead, a short broad nose, forward-facing nostrils, large ears, a large open mouth and small, widely spaced teeth. Increased fatty tissue in the forearms, large hands and tapering fingers, lax ligaments leading to flat feet and spinal and chest abnormalities occur. Life expectancy is probably near normal. Behavioural characteristics are largely unknown. Depression and schizophrenia have been reported in association with the disorder and in female carriers. Affected men usually have severe learning disabilities. Drop attacks and sleep apnoea syndrome have been reported. Further information may be obtained at www.clsf.info.

Coffin–Siris syndrome

The genetics of this disorder are unclear. The full syndrome occurs only in males, but female relatives may have learning disability and finger abnormalities. Physical features include sparse scalp hair and hirsutism affecting other parts of the body, especially the face and the back. The eyebrows may be joined, and other facial features include thick lips, a flat nasal bridge and a large mouth. Abnormalities of the finger- and toenails (especially the fifth fingernail), occasionally shortening of digits, hypotonia and joint laxity may also occur. The physical features vary in severity from one individual to another. Life expectancy depends largely on the severity of the physical features. Situation-specific maladaptive behaviours and autistic disorders have been reported, but there is no clear pattern of associated behaviours.

de Lange syndrome (Cornelia de Lange syndrome, Brachman de Lange syndrome)

This syndrome is believed to occur in about 1 in 60 000 live births, although some authors believe it to be more common. Mutations in a large gene on chromosome 5, the nipped B-like or NIPBL gene (named because its function resembles that of a fruit fly gene that produces a nipped wing) have been demonstrated in about 40% of people with the syndrome.

Affected individuals show growth retardation, distinctive facial features consisting of well-defined arched eyebrows which meet in the middle, long curled eyelashes, a small nose with forward-facing nostrils, a down-turned mouth with thin lips, and limb abnormalities such as small or shortened limbs, especially the arms. Hearing impairments, gut malformations and congenital heart defects also occur. The early mortality rate is high because of feeding problems, with regurgitation and vomiting leading to aspiration pneumonia in some cases. One study reported people surviving to their fifth decade.

Self-injury, autistic features and pleasurable responses to vestibular stimulation (e.g. spinning in a chair) have been reported as part of the behavioural repertoire. The degree of learning disability is usually severe, and speech is often very limited. However, some affected people have IQs within the normal range. Clinicians should be alert to the presence of pain and discomfort resulting from gastro-oesophageal reflux and other gastrointestinal abnormalities. Further information may be obtained at www.cdlsusa.org.

Cri du chat syndrome (CDCS, 5p-syndrome)

The prevalence of this syndrome is about 1 in 35 000 births. The short arm of chromosome 5 has a terminal deletion. The deletions vary in size, but the critical region for cri du chat syndrome is thought to be 5p15.2. In infancy there are feeding difficulties and the cry is abnormally high-pitched (cat-like, hence 'cri du chat'), but this is not an invariable or pathognomonic feature. The gene that causes the abnormal (cat-like) cry has been located at 15p13. It is therefore possible for affected babies with small deletions to have a cat-like cry but no other features of CDCS, or features of CDCS without the characteristic cry. Most deletions (about 85%) arise spontaneously, and the majority are of paternal origin. Around 15% of affected individuals have an unbalanced translocation, and in these cases the clinical features depend on the other chromosome involved. Less than 1% of cases are due to inherited deletions, which are usually very small.

Characteristic features are a round face, widely spaced slanting eyes, a small head, a broad flat nose, a small lower jaw and ear abnormalities. Larger deletions are associated with more pronounced clinical features, such as lower intelligence, smaller stature, lower weight and smaller head, as are translocations. The face often lengthens with development. and may be asymmetrical. Cleft lip or palate, curved fingers, hernias and orthopaedic abnormalities may occur. Older individuals often have premature greying of the hair. Life expectancy depends on the severity of the condition.

Hyperactivity is a problem for a substantial proportion of children, but may improve with age. Language development is often markedly delayed. The IQ associated with the syndrome ranged from 6 to 85 in one study. Further information may be obtained at www.criduchat.asn.au.

Duchenne muscular dystrophy

The prevalence of this condition at birth is about 1 in 4000 male births. This is an X-linked recessive condition in which deletions, duplications and mutations at Xp21 lead to failure to produce dystrophin, a protein component of muscle tissue. New mutations account for about 30% of cases. The syndrome is characterised by progressive muscle weakness, affecting the pelvis, upper leg and upper arm muscles first, with an onset typically between 2 and 6 years of age. Respiratory muscles are involved later in the disease process. Heart muscle abnormalities may also occur. The affected individual may need a wheelchair, usually at around 11 years of age, and death occurs in early adulthood, typically in the mid-twenties. Low mood, anxiety and social abnormalities are often problems, and may become more prominent as the disorder advances. These features may be normal reactions to a chronic and progressive physical disease. Specific learning disabilities are common, especially specific reading disorder. About 25% of those affected have a learning disability. Performance IQ is typically higher than verbal IQ. Further information may be obtained at www.mda.org.au.

18q syndrome

More than 100 cases of people with this syndrome have been described. The male:female ratio is 2:3. The deletion occurs spontaneously in about 80% of cases, and the break point is often at 18q21.2.

Physical features include an abnormally shaped skull, underdevelopment of the middle portion of the face, lip and nose abnormalities, small teeth, ear and eye abnormalities, and typically a squint and/or abnormal eye movements. Kyphosis, scoliosis, dimples over the joints and underdeveloped sexual organs in males have also been reported. In about 10% of cases death occurs within months of birth, but most affected people live to adulthood. Hyperactivity and aggressive behaviours have been documented, as have autistic and psychotic disorders. A husky voice is frequently reported. About 50% of reported cases have an IQ of between 30 and 70, with about 25% having IQs below 30 and 25% with IQs above 70. Language abnormalities are said to be common.

Lesch–Nyhan syndrome

The prevalence of this syndrome at birth is estimated to be between 1 in 100 000 and 1 in 1 000 000. It is an X-linked syndrome, and the disease results from a deficiency of a purine salvage enzyme, hypoxanthine-guanine phosphoribosyl transferase (HGPRT), which leads to hyperuricaemia and neurological disorder. Partial HGPRT deficiency results in gout. HGPRT is a 217-amino-acid peptide coded for by one gene that is divided into nine exons, located on the X chromosome at Xq26q27. Many different genetic lesions can cause HGPRT deficiency. Several complete and partial deletions, insertions and duplications of exons have been reported. Most lesions appear to be point mutations. Affected males may have had spontaneous mutations or inherited mutations from asymptomatic female carriers. Carrier detection and prenatal diagnosis are possible.

Neurological features include athetoid and other abnormal movements and spasticity. Growth retardation is usual. The presentation is usually with hypotonia and motor delay at about 4 months of age. Extrapyramidal signs (e.g. spasticity and choreo-athetoid movements) develop at about 9 months. Hyperreflexia and clonus appear at about 1 year. Dystonic movements may also develop, and dysarthria is common. Affected individuals may survive to the second or third decade of life. Death is usually due to kidney failure secondary to uric acid deposition or infection.

Compulsive severe self-injury occurs in over 85% of cases, and usually consists of finger and lip biting, with self-splinting in an attempt to prevent the behaviour. Other compulsive behaviours occur, including apparently compulsive aggressive acts. The mean age at onset of self-injury is 3.5 years, with wide variation. The IQ is usually between 40 and 80, but dysarthria and neurological problems limit the validity of standard IQ tests. Further information may be obtained at www.lndinfo.org.

Mucopolysaccharidoses

The mucopolysaccharide group of disorders has both names (Hunter syndrome, Hurler syndrome, Sanfillipo syndrome, Morquio syndrome and Schie syndrome) and numerical designations (MPS IIA/B, MPS IH, MPS IIIA/B/C/D, MPS IVA/B and MPS IS, respectively). The disorders result from deficiencies in enzyme systems involved in the degradation of glycosaminoglycans, leading to the accumulation of abnormal metabolic products.

All of these syndromes are rare disorders. The incidence among liveborn children is approximately 1 in 100 000 for Hunter and Hurler syndromes, 1 in 200 000 for Sanfillipo syndrome and Morquio syndrome and 1 in 500 000 for Schie syndrome. The transmission is autosomal recessive except in Hunter syndrome (IIA and IIB), which is X-linked. Physical features vary. Coarse facial features ('gargoylism'), hepatosplenomegaly, joint stiffness, eye abnormalities and short stature occur in many of the disorders. Life expectancy varies from death in the first decade in Hurler syndrome through survival into the second or third decade in Sanfillipo syndrome, to survival to adult life in Hunter syndrome and Schie syndrome.

Sleep problems and abnormal nocturnal behaviours such as staying up all night, night-time laughing and singing, sudden crying out and chewing of bedclothes have been reported in association with Sanfillipo syndrome, and have been shown to respond to behavioural management strategies. Cognitive abilities range from normal intelligence in Schie syndrome to severe learning disability and progressive cognitive deterioration in Hurler syndrome. SanfilIipo syndrome is associated with slower progressive cognitive impairment than that seen in Hurler syndrome, but often with marked behavioural and psychiatric abnormalities consistent with the diagnosis of childhood disintegrative disorder. Further information may be obtained at www.mpssociety.org.

Myotonic dystrophy

Myotonic dystrophy affects about 1 in 8000 liveborn infants and is an autosomal dominant condition with the responsible gene localised to chromosome 19 (there is an increase in cytosine–thymine–guanine (CTG) trinucleotide repeats within the non-coding portion of the myoprotein kinase gene). Anticipation (an increase in severity of symptoms and an earlier age at onset) has been observed in many families, and probably results from an increase in the number of repeats (see the above section on fragile X syndrome for a discussion of a similar genetic process).

Physical features involve muscle weakness and wasting. Facial weakness results in ptosis (drooping eyelids) and a 'slack' jaw. Men often have a characteristic pattern of hair loss. A failure of muscle relaxation after use causes speech and swallowing difficulties. Cataracts are common, as are cardiac conduction problems. Particular care is needed if a general anaesthetic is required. Death most commonly occurs in the sixth decade. Personality abnormalities and affective symptoms have been reported, and learning disability occurs in a substantial minority of affected people. Further information may be obtained at www.myotonicdystrophy.org.

Neurofibromatosis type I (von Recklinghausen's disease)

This autosomal dominant disorder occurs in about 1 in 3000 births. The gene responsible is localised to 17q11.2. The gene product, neurofibromin, is thought to suppress tumour formation by regulating cell division. A high spontaneous mutation rate means that about 50% of all cases arise in unaffected families.

Tumours develop from the connective tissue of nerve sheaths. Two or more of the following features are usually required for diagnosis: six or more café-au-lait (light brown) skin lesions; two or more neurofibromas or one plexiform neurofibroma (tumours of the nerve sheath); freckling of the groin or armpit; lisch nodules; an optic nerve glioma (tumour); a bony lesion characteristic of neurofibromatosis; a first-degree relative with the disorder. Life expectancy depends on the nature and severity of the clinical features.

About 50% of affected children have speech or language abnormalities. Distractibility and impulsiveness may be problems. Learning disability is present in around 10% of affected individuals. Specific developmental disorders such as difficulties with reading, writing or numeracy affect about 50% of these children. Visuo-spatial abnormalities and lack of co-ordination have also been described. Further information can be obtained at www.geneclinics.org/profiles/nf1.

Phenylketonuria

Classical phenylketonuria (PKU) affects about 1 in 10 000 liveborn children in the UK. Other hyperphenylalaninaemias also occur. The disorder results from a deficiency of the enzyme phenylalanine hydroxylase. The extent of the deficiency varies, with a spectrum of resulting clinical conditions ranging from classical phenylketonuria to benign hyperphenylalaninaemia. The gene that regulates phenylalanine hydroxylase is located on the long arm of chromosome 12 at 12q22-24.1, and is subject to various mutations. The classical form is inherited in an autosomal recessive manner. Prenatal diagnosis and the detection of hetero-zygotes with one defective copy of the gene are possible. About 2% of cases are due to a deficiency of tetrahydrobiopterin rather than phenylalanine hydroxylase.

Physical features include blond hair, blue eyes, eczema, an unusual 'mouse-like' body odour, microcephaly in 50% of cases, epilepsy in 25% of cases, and tremor and movement disorders or spasticity. Life expectancy depends on the response to dietary restriction of phenylalanine and the presence of complications. In the UK all newborns are screened for the disorder. A low-phenylalanine diet is usually continued through childhood. There is some debate about the age at which it is appropriate to lift or relax dietary restrictions. Amino-acid supplements may be used to block phenylalanine uptake. Dietary control is essential when affected women become pregnant, because hyperphenylalaninaemia is toxic to the fetus, leading to learning disability, microcephaly, and facial and heart abnormalities.

Untreated phenylketonuria is associated with a number of maladaptive behaviours and behavioural syndromes, including overactivity, self-injury and autism. Autism and many of the other features do not occur in children managed with low-phenylalanine diets. Those who have not been treated may have moderate to profound learning disabilities, irritability and marked social impair-ments. Inadequate dietary control is associated with deficits in mathematical, visuo-spatial and language skills. Further information can be obtained at www.nspku.org.

Prader–Willi syndrome

The incidence is around 1 in 40 000 liveborn infants. About 70% of those affected have a deletion affecting the long arm of chromosome 15 (del 15q11q13), and the deleted chromosome is always of paternal origin. About 29% of cases have maternal uniparental disomy (both of the chromosome 15s are inherited from the mother, with no paternal chromosome 15) and about 1% have an imprinting error. This condition is thought to arise through the lack of a paternal contribu-tion to an area within 15q11q13.

Infants are hypotonic or floppy and have feeding problems associated with a failure to suck. Many will have been tube fed. In early childhood there is a switch to marked overeating. Affected adults are of short stature and have small hands and feet, a characteristic pattern of facial appearance and a lack of sexual development. Many are obese as a result of the relative lack of satiety leading to overeating. There is an increased prevalence of curvature of the spine or scoliosis as well as other orthopaedic abnormalities, and diabetes or heart failure may result from obesity. Life expectancy depends on the severity of obesity. Most of those affected die before the sixth decade, but this situation may improve with early diagnosis and improved dietary management. A woman aged 71 years with del 15q11q13 has been reported. The commonest cause of death is heart failure.

Affected individuals have an almost insatiable appetite. They may steal food and consume 'unpalatable' food such as rotting or frozen food or pet food. A variety of sleep abnormalities and a lowering of the threshold for loss of temper are seen in these people. About 80% of cases pick or scratch their skin. Insistence on routines, obsessional behaviours and psychoses have also been reported. Anecdotal reports suggest that the pain threshold may be raised.

About 5% of individuals with this syndrome have overall cognitive abilities with IQs in excess of 85, 27% have borderline cognitive abilities with IQs between 70 and 85, and the incidence of mild, moderate, severe and profound learning disability is 34%, 27%, 5% and less than 1%, respectively. There are deficits in auditory information processing, and relative strengths in visuo-spatial tasks. Further information can be obtained at www.ipwso.org.

Rett syndrome

Rett syndrome, which causes significant learning disabilities in women, has a prevalence estimated at 1 in 10 000 women. The syndrome results from a mutation in the MeCP2 gene located at Xq28. The mutation was considered to be lethal in males, but there are a small number of men with the syndrome. The severity of the syndrome in women depends on the percentage of cells with the normal MeCP2 gene active after X inactivation. If more of the X chromosomes with normal MeCP2 gene have been inactivated, the syndrome is likely to be more severe.

The affected child appears normal at birth. For the first 12 months no major abnormalities are apparent, although the child may be placid, lack muscle tone and be relatively immobile. They acquire skills up to about 1 year of age, but regression begins at around 18 months, with loss of skills, especially speech and use of the hands. The incidence of physical disorders increases with age, and these include scoliosis, spasticity and leg deformities. Epilepsy is common. Pathological changes include a reduction in brain size with reduced cortical thickness, reduced neuronal branching, and depigmentation of the basal ganglia. Many affected girls reach adulthood, but about 1% of them die each year, early death being associated with increased physical disability.

Sleep disturbance, withdrawal and episodes of crying occur during the phase of regression at around 18 months of age. This phase is followed by a developmental plateau, when extreme agitation and over-breathing interspersed with episodes of cessation of breathing become apparent. The most prominent feature of the behavioural phenotype is the presence of stereotyped movements, especially midline 'hand-wringing' movements. Affected women and girls usually have profound learning disability. Further information can be obtained at www.rettsyndrome.org.uk.

Rubinstein–Taybi syndrome

This syndrome is one of the 25 commonest multiple congenital anomaly syndromes seen in genetic clinics in the USA, and it has an estimated incidence of 1 in 125 000 liveborn infants. Recent studies have found small deletions at 16p13.3 in about 25% of cases. A few apparently familial cases have been reported, and four sets of concordant monozygotic (i.e. identical) twins have been reported.

The affected individuals are usually short, and have a small head, a beaked or straight nose and downward slanting eyes. They have a stiff gait and their thumbs and first toes have broad terminal phalanges (ends), often with an angulation deformity. Other congenital anomalies are not uncommon. Inadequate weight gain in infancy, congenital heart defects, urinary tract abnormalities and severe constipation contribute to morbidity, and this is reflected in a hospitalisation rate 10 times higher than that of the general population. Affected people can survive to the seventh decade.

Findings from postal questionnaire surveys in the USA and UK indicate that people with this syndrome have a friendly, happy disposition, a propensity to self-stimulatory activities such as rocking, and an intolerance of loud noises. Rocking, spinning and hand flapping were found to be common in the UK survey. A survey of non-institutionalised children reported an average IQ of 51. Another report stated that 75% of affected individuals had an IQ of less than 50. Carers reported a short attention span in 90% of a sample of 41 people with the syndrome in the UK. Further information can be obtained at www.rubinstein-taybi.org.

Smith–Lemli–Opitz syndrome

This syndrome is thought to occur in about 1 in 30 000 live births. Mild cases may be undiagnosed and the syndrome may be relatively common, as it is said to be one of the commonest autosomal recessive conditions affecting people of White European origin in North America. It appears to be three times more common in men than in women, but this may be due to the fact that the sexual abnormalities are easier to detect in men. It is an autosomal recessive condition in which a deficiency of the enzyme 7-dehydrocholesterol reductase results in elevated levels of a cholesterol precursor.

During pregnancy, the fetus may show growth retardation. Affected individuals have a small head, drooping eyelids, a squint, forward-facing nostrils, a small lower jaw and finger abnormalities such as extra fingers and fusing together of fingers. Males have abnormalities of their external genitalia, such as small testes or penis, abnormal opening of the ureter (e.g. hypospadia), undescended testes and female genitalia. Cleft palate and abnormalities of almost all major organ systems may also occur. Life expectancy depends on the severity of associated features. Some severely affected infants die shortly after birth, but mildly affected adults probably have near-normal life expectancy.

There is little information available about behavioural and cognitive characteristics. Intelligence ranges from normal to severe learning disability. One report describes aggressive and self-injurious behaviours in an affected girl. Further information can be obtained at www.geneclinics.org/profiles/slo.

Smith–Magenis syndrome

This syndrome, which occurs in about 1 in 50 000 births, is associated with deletions at 17p11.2. Affected individuals have a flattened mid-face, an abnormally shaped upper lip, short hands and feet, a single transverse palmar crease, abnormally shaped or placed ears and occasionally a high arched palate or a protruding tongue. The facial features coarsen with development. Ear and eye disorders such as otitis media and squint are relatively common. The life expectancy of affected individuals is probably near normal, and a 65-year-old with the syndrome has been described.

Newborn babies with the syndrome are usually placid, 'floppy' and feed with difficulty. This changes to hyperactivity and self-injury (e.g. head banging, pulling out finger and toe nails and the insertion of objects into body orifices) from about 18 months onwards. Self-hugging and mid-line hand clapping have been reported in a series of cases. Sleep disorders are common, with some children waking repeatedly in a state of agitation. An absence of rapid eye movement (REM) sleep has been reported in some patients. Many affected children appear to be relatively insensitive to pain. Those with the syndrome usually have moderate learning disability. The severity of the cognitive impairment is correlated with the size of the 17p11 deletion. Speech delay is more pronounced than delay in motor achievements. Further information can be obtained at www.prisms.org.

Sotos syndrome (cerebral gigantism)

First described by Sotos in 1964, this syndrome is characterised by excessively rapid growth, acromegalic features and a non-progressive cerebral disorder with mental retardation. Mutation of the NSD1 gene mapped to 5q35 has been reported in children with the syndrome. Reported cases have included familial and sporadic ones.

Affected individuals have distinctive facial features consisting of a round face and forehead, a prominent jaw, anteverted nasal opening and slanting eye fissures. There is a period of growth acceleration in early childhood with advanced bone age, developmental delay and motor clumsiness. Constipation is common, and drooling may be a problem. About 50% of cases have seizures, sometimes confined to febrile convulsions, but occasionally the epilepsy is difficult to treat. Respiratory tract infections lead to a vulnerability to conductive hearing loss. There is no information available on life expectancy, although some authors suggest that physical and behavioural abnormalities become less pronounced with development and that life expectancy may be near normal.

Behavioural problems are common in the cases reported, and include aggressive and destructive behaviours, unhappiness and poor social relationships. Early feeding problems with reluctance to chew have been described, as have obsessive-compulsive symptoms, temper tantrums, pica, excessive eating and obesity and sleep abnormalities. Some authors have suggested that behavioural abnormalities are perceived as being more severe in children with Sotos syndrome because of their large size. Cognitive abilities range from above average intelligence to severe learning disability. Some children have specific learning problems. Speech abnormalities include echolalia and perseveration (inability to 'move on' in speech). Verbal IQs tend to increase with age, whereas performance IQ tends to remain constant or decrease. Overactivity and attention deficit have also been described. Further information can be obtained at www.well.com/user/sssa.

Tuberous sclerosis

The incidence is about 1 in 7000. It is an autosomal dominant condition, but up to 80% of cases arise as a result of spontaneous mutations. The disorder is genetically heterogeneous, with gene linkage to 9q34 and 16p13. The physical features are very variable. The previously used 'diagnostic triad' of epilepsy, mental retardation and a characteristic facial skin lesion is no longer considered helpful, as it is seen in only about 30% of individuals with the disease. Tuberous sclerosis is a multi-system disorder, with hamartomatous tumours (arising from primitive cells) affecting the brain in 90% of cases, the skin in 96% of cases, the kidneys in 60%, the heart in 50%, and the eyes in 47% of cases, as well as the teeth, bones, lungs and other organs. About 80% of affected people have epilepsy. Life expectancy depends on the location and the number of lesions. Brain tumours and kidney lesions are common causes of death.

Tuberous sclerosis is associated with autism and related disorders, hyperactivity and attention deficit disorder, obsessive and ritualistic behaviours, sleep problems, and occasionally self-injurious or aggressive behaviours. Less than 50% of affected people have a learning disability. Attention deficit is common. Of those with learning disability, a high proportion have an IQ of less than 30. Further information can be obtained at www.tuberous-sclerosis.org.

Velo-cardio-facial syndrome

This condition is associated with microdeletions at 22q11. Physical features include cardiac anomalies (such as ventriculoseptal defects, pulmonary stenosis and cardiac outlet abnormalities), facial dysmorphology with a prominent nose with broad bridge and squared tip, a small head and/or a small lower jaw, ocular abnormalities in a proportion of cases and cleft palate, short stature and long thin hyperextensible fingers. Life expectancy depends primarily on the severity of the heart abnormalities.

Affected individuals show abnormalities of social behaviour. A high prevalence of personality disorders and psychotic disorders during adolescence and early adult life has been reported in some studies. Over 90% of cases have a learning disability, and language problems are common. Further information can be obtained at www.vcfsef.org.

Williams' syndrome (idiopathic infantile hypercalcaemia)

The syndrome affects between 1 in 25 000 and 1 in 50 000 liveborn infants. Most cases are sporadic, although a few familial cases have been reported where the transmission seems to be autosomal dominant. The syndrome is at least in part due to gene deletion of the WS critical region that encompasses the elastin gene at 7q11.3.

Infants have difficulties in feeding, are irritable, have constipation and fail to thrive. Over 60% of affected children have a high level of calcium, which responds to treatment with a low-calcium diet and vitamin D restriction. The face is distinctive, with prominent cheeks, a wide mouth and a flat nasal bridge (often described as 'elfin-like'). Kidney and heart lesions (especially supravalvular aortic stenosis and peripheral pulmonary artery stenosis) are common, and growth is usually retarded. Life expectancy is related to metabolic and heart abnormalities.

Social disinhibition with abnormal friendliness towards strangers, overactivity, poor concentration, eating and sleeping abnormalities, abnormal anxiety, poor peer relationships and abnormally sensitive hearing have been reported. Around

95% of children with the disorder have a moderate or severe learning disability. Verbal abilities are better developed than visuo-spatial and motor skills. There is an unusual command of language – expressive language is superficially fluent and articulate, but verbose. Comprehension is far more limited. Further information can be obtained at www.williams-syndrome.org.

Sex chromosome anomalies

Klinefelter syndrome

The prevalence of this syndrome at birth is between 1 in 5000 and 1 in 1000 live male births. This is a disorder caused by a surplus of X chromosomes in phenotypic males. Two-thirds of cases have a 47 XXY chromosome complement. Height, weight and head circumference are below average at birth. Increased growth, especially of the legs, occurs from 3 years of age onwards. Affected men are usually taller than their fathers, but head size remains small. Puberty normally occurs, but testosterone production falls in early adulthood. Affected adults have a normal-sized penis but small testes. About 60% of cases have some breast enlargement. Life expectancy is thought to be normal.

Boys with XXY are typically introverted and less assertive and sociable than other children, with poorer school performance. Adults may show increased rates of antisocial behaviour and impulsiveness. The IQ distribution is skewed downward, although measured full-scale IQs run from around 60 to over 130. Performance scores usually exceed verbal scores. Most affected children receive speech and language therapy, and expressive language deficits are often more pronounced than problems with receptive language. Further information can be obtained at www.klinefeltersyndrome.org.

Turner syndrome

This syndrome affects about 1 in 2500 live female births. The abnormality is much more common at conception, but about 99% of affected fetuses are miscarried. The genetic abnormality is the loss or abnormality of one X chromosome in women. About 50% of cases have an XO chromosome complement, although a very small proportion of normal cell lines may be present, and about 40% have mosaicism. Around 15% of cases have a 45,XO/46,XX karyotype.

Affected children have a short stature in childhood. Ovarian failure occurs before birth, and puberty does not occur naturally. Dysmorphic features include a webbed neck, a low hairline at the rear of the head, widely spaced nipples and multiple pigmented naevi. Around 20% of affected women have an abnormality of the large artery emerging from the heart. Life expectancy is believed to be normal.

Hyperactivity and distractibility are common in childhood. Poor social skills and social withdrawal may be problems in later childhood and adolescence. Immaturity and problems in peer relationships have also been reported. One study found that about 25% of girls with the syndrome had psychiatric disorders of a severity comparable with that of cases referred for treatment. The women usually have normal IQs, but specific cognitive abnormalities are frequently found, including a relative deficit in performance skills, and depression of Wechsler sub-test scores for items such as Block Design, Object Assembly, Arithmetic and Information. Some verbal measures, such as verbal recognition and the use of advanced vocabulary, are typically enhanced. This may lead to an overestimation of abilities. There is considerable variation in cognitive profile between affected women. Further information can be obtained at www.tss.org.uk.

XXX syndrome

This syndrome has an incidence of about 1 in 1000 female births. Most cases are not diagnosed. There is a primary non-disjunction of a maternal or paternal X chromosome. 48 XXXX is much rarer, and only about 40 cases have been reported. Newborn babies have a low birth weight and small head circumference. Height in adult life is usually increased. Fertility is unimpaired, but there may be deficits in balance or fine motor coordination. Life expectancy is thought to be normal.

Underactivity and withdrawal have been reported, and emotional development may be slowed. Most individuals with this syndrome appear to adapt to adult life without difficulties. Women with the syndrome usually have IQs of between 80 and 90. Women with XXXX syndrome have lower IQs (55–75). An expressive language delay is typical. In some cases there is a relatively poor short-term auditory memory. Further information can be obtained at www.triplo-x.org.

XYY syndrome

This condition has an incidence of about 1 in 1000 live male births. There is a primary non-disjunction of the Y chromosome. About 10% of cases have mosaic 46,XY/47,XYY chromosome complement. Offspring rarely have two Y chromosomes. Affected individuals show an increase in body and leg length between 4 and 9 years of age. Most are over 10 cm taller than their fathers as adults. Sexual development and fertility are unaffected. Balance and coordination may be minimally compromised. Life expectancy is normal.

Distractibility, hyperactivity and temper tantrums appear to be relatively common in childhood. Speech and language problems are common. Overactivity and distractibility may lead to educational problems. IQ is usually lower than that of siblings, but only just below population means.

Further information

Information about individual syndromes is available from the source mentioned after each syndrome in the text above. The *Contact a Family Directory of Specific Conditions and Rare Disorders (CaF Directory)* is widely used as a source of basic information about characteristics and carer organisations. A new paper edition is published in January each year, and it is also available in CD-ROM format on a quarterly subscription basis (www.cafamily.org.uk).

References

Britto JA, Moore RL, Evans RD, *et al.* (2001) Negative autoregulation of fibroblast growth factor receptor 2 expression characterizing cranial development in cases of Apert (P253R mutation) and Pfeiffer (C278F mutation) syndromes and suggesting a basis for differences in their cranial phenotypes. *J Neurosurg*. 95: 660–73.

Koshino T, Lalande M and Wagstaff J (1997) UBE3A/E6-AP mutations cause Angelman syndrome. *Nat Genet*. **15**: 70–3.

Further reading

O'Brien G (ed.) (2002) *Behavioural Phenotypes in Clinical Practice*. MacKeith Press, Cambridge, MA.

Chapter 7

Physical health problems in people with intellectual disabilities

Verinder Prasher and Ashok Roy

Introduction

Healthcare provision for people with learning disabilities has, until recently, received little attention. During the early part of this century, when a eugenic view prevailed, children with learning disabilities were often admitted to long-stay institutions and their heathcare needs were neglected. With the recent increase in public awareness of health issues, support from the Government with the publication of *The Health of the Nation* (Department of Health 1995) and greater advocacy, there is now the potential for much needed change. At present, most causes of learning disabilities (e.g. chromosome abnormalities or birth trauma) are untreatable. However, high-quality healthcare may reduce the impact of disabilities or handicaps and improve quality of life.

The closure of large institutions, the advent of care in the community and the greater role of primary care teams led by general practitioners have increased the number of people with learning disabilities living in the community either in supported group homes or with their families. They now live longer as a result of improvements in healthcare. This in turn has led to an increase in the number of older people with learning disabilities, who have medical problems related to ageing as well as problems associated with the cause of their learning problem.

Several researchers have demonstrated a high prevalence of untreated physical disorders in people with learning disabilities (Van Schrojenstein Lantman-de Valk *et al.* 2000), in particular in the older population (Moss *et al.* 1993). The commonest forms of pathology include visual impairment, hearing loss, dental disease, musculoskeletal problems, endocrine disorders, epilepsy and obesity (Prasher 1994). The majority of people with learning disabilities living in the community have been reported to have one or more chronic physical and/or mental disorders (i.e. sufficient to warrant ongoing medical intervention) (Cohen 2001).

Common physical health problems and related issues are discussed in this chapter. Phenotypic characteristics of syndromes that cause learning disabilities are addressed in Chapter 6, and psychiatric disorders are discussed in Chapter 3.

Excess weight and obesity

Obesity is said to be present when there is an excessive amount of body fat. However, criteria for deciding what is 'excessive', and the accurate measurement of fat (adipose tissue), remain controversial. Body mass index (BMI) (weight in kilograms, divided by height in metres squared), is widely used as an indicator of the severity of obesity. The division by height squared makes allowance for height, and increases the value of BMI as an indicator of obesity in people of short stature (sometimes a feature of disorders that cause learning disabilities). BMI is conventionally divided into the following bands:

- < 20, underweight
- 20–24.9, desirable
- 25–29.9, overweight
- 30–34.9, obesity
- 35–39.9, medically significant obesity
- 40–44.9, super obesity
- ≥ 45, morbid obesity.

Among adults (age 16–65 years) in the general population, 34% of men and 24% of women are overweight and 6% of men and 8% of women are obese (BMI of ≥ 30). Obesity is most prevalent in middle age, has a significant hereditary component and is more common among people from lower socio-economic groups. Obesity may sometimes result from the development of an endocrine disorder, or be associated with the use of certain drugs (e.g. steroids and oral contraceptives).

Obesity is common among people with learning disabilities, and may be associated with particular syndromes such as Down syndrome and Prader–Willi syndrome. Prevalence rates for being overweight are in the range 16–49% for men and 21–63% for women with learning disabilities. Rates for obesity are in the range 16–20% for men and 17–25% for women. In adults with Down syndrome, 31% of men and 22% of women were recently reported to be overweight, while 48% of men and 47% of women were reported to be obese (Prasher 1995).

The influence of severity of learning disabilities and place of residence on obesity has been investigated. The highest rates of obesity are found in people living at home, followed by those living in group homes, with the lowest rates being found among individuals living in institutions. The reasons for increased obesity in people living at home are unclear, but may include access to food and relative underactivity. The effect of severity of learning disabilities remains controversial, with some studies showing a low rate of obesity in people with severe learning disabilities while others have found no association. The cause of obesity is unknown, but is probably multi-factorial, involving calorie intake, decreased resting metabolic rate, sedentary lifestyle, endocrine abnormalities (e.g. hypothyroidism), hypotonia (muscle 'floppiness') and possibly the presence of extra genetic material in some syndromes. Obesity often starts in childhood and is maintained in later life.

Obesity is associated with increased mortality (death rate) and morbidity (rate of physical disease), and has a detrimental effect on the quality of life of affected individuals. Diseases and disorders associated with obesity include coronary heart disease, gallstones, hypertension, diabetes, gout and arthritis.

The management of obesity in people with learning disabilities is therefore of considerable importance. A reduction in weight can only be achieved by decreasing energy intake or increasing output, or a combination of the two. Weight-reducing diets and exercise have been shown to reduce obesity in the general population, although motivation and support are often crucial in determining whether such strategies are successful. Few studies have addressed the management of obesity in people with learning disabilities (Stewart *et al.* 1994). Treatments that have been suggested include social reinforcement, self-recording and multi-component treatment programmes. The role of drug treatments (appetite suppressants or stimulants such as fenfluramine, or hormonal treatments such as thyroxine) and surgical intervention in people with learning disabilities is limited. Prevention remains the most important strategy.

Heart disease

Congenital heart abnormalities are not uncommon in babies with learning disabilities. Abnormalities are particularly associated with Down syndrome, Cornelia de Lange syndrome, cri du chat syndrome and Turner's syndrome. Although heart abnormalities are usually diagnosed in childhood, individuals may live until adulthood, when such pathology may cause complications. Furthermore, new lesions may develop in adulthood (e.g. prolapse of the mitral valve). Table 7.1 lists some common heart problems seen in people with learning disabilities.

In adulthood, pulmonary artery hypertension and pulmonary vascular obstructive disease in association with congestive heart failure are major complications of childhood cardiac defects. Children with known heart disease should be followed up closely into adulthood for evidence of heart failure or pulmonary complications. The accurate diagnosis of any resulting disease may be difficult, and referral to a cardiologist may be necessary.

The rise in blood pressure with age which is apparent in the general population has not been adequately investigated in people with learning disabilities. In people with Down syndrome, several studies have commented on the presence of a lower mean blood pressure than is found in the general population (Richards and Enver 1979). Such findings suggest that people with Down syndrome are less at risk of hypertension, myocardial infarction and cerebrovascular accidents. The risk is further reduced by the low prevalence of smoking in this population. Further research is needed into the prevalence of hypertension and its complications in adults with learning disabilities as a whole.

Table 7.1 Types of cardiac disorders

Congenital	Acquired
Aortic coarctation	Arrhythmias
Hypoplastic ventricle	Cardiac failure
Ventricular septal defects	Ischaemic heart disease
Patent ductus arteriosus	Hypertension
Tetralogy of Fallot	
Subaortic stenosis	
Atrial septal defect	

Symptoms suggestive of heart disease include breathlessness, swelling of the ankles, cyanotic episodes, feeding difficulties, chest pain, palpitations, fainting and tiredness. Signs found on physical examination include fast and/or irregular pulse, abnormal heart sounds, the presence of a heart murmur, and high or low blood pressure. A number of investigations, including electrocardiography, chest X-ray and echocardiography, can aid diagnosis.

Assessment for cardiovascular morbidity is imperative whenever a person with learning disabilities shows signs of distress or decline in functioning. For example, heart failure may first be noticed as a result of its effects, which can include a loss of skills or behavioural change. The latter may give the impression that the person has a psychiatric condition.

Disorders of the respiratory tract

Structural abnormalities of the airways involving the nasal passages, oropharynx and lungs have all been described in people with learning disabilities. There may be abnormalities of the ribs or rib-cage with an increased prevalence of pectus excavatum (funnel chest) and pectus carinatum (pigeon chest). As with cardiac problems, abnormalities may be detected in childhood and may persist into adulthood.

Respiratory tract infections such as acute and chronic bronchitis cause significant morbidity and mortality in people with learning disabilities, despite the use of antibiotics. This is particularly important after surgery. Pneumonia remains one of the major causes of death in people with learning disabilities. Chronic rhinitis (persistent runny nose) may appear not to be too serious, but can nevertheless cause considerable persistent problems.

Common symptoms of respiratory disease include cough, purulent sputum, bloodstained sputum, chest pain, breathlessness, wheeze and cyanosis. On examination, abnormal breath sounds, discoloration of the fingers and chest wall tenderness may be found. Further investigations, including microbiological and cytological examination of sputum, blood examination, chest X-ray, bronchoscopy and lung biopsy, may be required.

Treatment involves supportive care, maintaining fluid intake, oxygen, antibiotics, physiotherapy and possibly diuretics and bronchodilators. The presence of congenital heart disease may lead to pulmonary artery hypertension with subsequent respiratory failure.

Obstructive sleep apnoea has been associated with people with learning disabilities, and in particular with Down syndrome. Obstructive sleep apnoea occurs when respiratory airflow from the upper airways to the lungs is impeded, usually for 10 seconds or more, resulting in low levels of oxygen in the blood (hypoxaemia) or elevated levels of carbon dioxide in the blood (hypercarbia). During the interruption of airflow, respiration continues but airflow ceases, affecting pharyngeal dilator muscles, causing their relaxation and subsequent airway collapse. The cause of obstructive sleep apnoea is probably multi-factorial, involving anatomical, physiological and neurological aspects. Other ongoing respiratory abnormalities may worsen this condition. The symptoms of obstructive sleep apnoea include snoring, interrupted breathing during sleep, restless sleep, difficulty awakening, chronic nocturnal cough, daytime somnolence, mouth breathing, failure to thrive, morning headaches, behavioural changes, and school problems and developmental delay in children.

The diagnosis of obstructive sleep apnoea depends on the presence of the above symptoms, demonstrated by the carer tape recording the night-time sleeping and breathing patterns. If there is a suspicion that the condition is present, a referral to a respiratory chest physician for a full assessment is required to rule out any treatable causes. Treatment involves management of the acute airway obstruction with high-pressure oxygen, and possibly surgery to the upper respiratory tract. Non-surgical intervention, such as dieting and exercise, may also be beneficial.

The presence of significant respiratory pathology may present as a decline in functioning, and may also be misdiagnosed as a psychiatric disorder.

The gastrointestinal disorders

Abnormalities of the gastrointestinal tract are a common occurrence in people with learning disabilities. Common congenital abnormalities include pyloric stenosis, duodenal stenosis or atresia, imperforate anus, Hirschsprung's disease and malrotation.

As with other conditions, these are usually more common in infants and children than in adults. Gastro-oesophageal reflux may be present in adults and may subsequently lead to oesophageal strictures that require surgical intervention. Other conditions may continue into adulthood, leading to complications (e.g. chronic constipation in Hirschsprung's disease). With interventions from paediatricians, dietitians, surgeons and other professionals, many of the problems may be managed in the same way that they would be in the general population.

Symptoms of alimentary disease include discoloration of the skin, pain, loss of appetite, vomiting, heartburn, difficulty in swallowing, constipation, diarrhoea, loss of weight and bleeding. Investigations include blood tests, examination of stools, plain abdominal X-ray examination, barium studies, endoscopy and ultrasound studies.

Constipation may lead to disruptive behaviour and irritability. Loss of weight and appetite due to gastrointestinal pathology may be misdiagnosed as symptoms of depression. A screen for the possibility of abdominal pathology must therefore be made in all adults who show signs of being unwell.

Urinary tract disorders

Congenital abnormalities of the urinary system include hydronephrosis, obstructive uropathy, renal agenesis, etc. Such abnormalities may persist into adulthood, when secondary complications may arise (e.g. urinary tract infections, renal failure and hypertension). Symptoms of a urinary tract infection include increased frequency of urination, pain while passing urine and discoloration of urine. Investigations for possible kidney disease include examination of urinary volume and concentration, analysis for the presence of abnormal constituents (e.g. protein, blood, bacteria), blood tests, radiological tests, ultrasound examination and biopsy. Routine biochemical screening for renal function and routine urinalysis are recommended.

Disorders of the reproductive system

Anatomical and physiological abnormalities found in men include undescended testes on one or both sides, underdeveloped penis and scrotum, distal hypospadia and impaired sperm production. An undescended testis may result in infertility and an increased risk of a testicular tumour (Braun *et al.* 1985). Secondary sex characteristics develop but can be delayed. In women, ovarian hypoplasia, and hypertrophied labia majora but poorly developed labia minora may be found.

Most women with learning disabilities begin to menstruate between the ages of 10 and 14 years, but several cases of premature puberty have been reported, often associated with thyroid disorder. Problems such as menorrhagia, irregular bleeding, dysmenorrhoea and premenstrual syndrome can also occur in women with learning disabilities, although they may be more difficult to diagnose because of difficulties in communication (Wingfield *et al.* 1994). As endocrine disorders are common in women with learning disabilities, there may be secondary menstrual irregularities.

Recently, sexual awareness among people with learning disabilities and the need for gynaecological care have become a focus of concern. It is generally accepted that it is rare for women with learning disabilities to attend for gynaecological assessment. This is of considerable importance, as routine screening advocated for women in general, such as cervical smear screening and breast screening, is not often offered to women with a learning disability. Examination of the breast and of the pelvic region may be difficult, and greater care and considerable understanding and empathy are required for such examinations to be successful. Regular Well Woman checks are recommended, although issues of consent and privacy need to be borne in mind. A number of dilemmas exist with regard to screening of people who cannot consent. Sexuality and consent are considered in Chapter 10.

Neurological and skeletal aspects of health

Numerous neurological and musculoskeletal abnormalities have been reported in people with learning disabilities, in particular among those with cerebral palsy. These may range from general abnormalities of stature, gait, muscle tone, speech and limb movements to specific abnormalities (e.g. atlanto-axial instability). The majority of people with learning disabilities are of short stature, although specific syndromes may be associated with tall stature (e.g. Klinefelter's syndrome). Metabolic disorders of the bone (e.g. osteoporosis with loss of bone mass) may be seen in association with endocrine disorders, syndromes such as Hurler syndrome and Hunter syndrome (*see* Chapter 6) and drug therapy for epilepsy (e.g. phenytoin). Undetected osteoporosis may present as bone pain or spontaneous fractures. Other minor abnormalities such as collapsing flat feet may also contribute to disability.

Cerebral palsy is a persistent disorder of movement and posture caused by non-progressive damage to the developing brain. Many causes can lead to cerebral palsy, but the commonest factors include pre-term birth, brain malformations and convulsions at an early age.

There are several forms of cerebral palsy with differing neurological problems. The types of movement disorder are generally classified as hypotonic, ataxic, spastic, athetoid and tremulous. The limbs may be affected by pareses of varying degree and varying combinations (hemiplegia, paraplegia or quadriplegia). A large number of other neurological deficits may be present, depending on the site and type of brain damage. Muscular contractures may lead to dislocation of joints (e.g. dislocation of the hip joint) and may be a cause of pain and discomfort. Impairment of mobility, contractures, increased muscle tone and poor posture may cause considerable difficulties.

Clinical features of musculoskeletal disorders include joint pain, stiffness, swelling, reduced mobility and involvement of other systemic organs. Common problems in people with Down syndrome include subluxation and dislocation of the cervical spine, hip and patella. Cervical spine subluxation at the atlanto-occipital and atlanto-axial regions is one of the potentially most serious ortho-paedic conditions encountered in individuals with Down syndrome. They may present with local neck pain, muscle weakness, paralysis of the limbs and gait abnormalities. On examination there may be impaired mobility of the neck, head tilt, brisk deep tendon reflexes, extensor plantar responses and ankle clonus. A history of neck trauma can be elicited in many cases. Acute onset is more likely to respond to treatment than chronic symptomatology. Regular screening has been undertaken for people with this disorder, as asymptomatic individuals may become symptomatic, leading to spinal cord injury. X-ray imaging is recom-mended, although its reliability may be poor.

It may be necessary to restrict sporting activities such as training or competitive gymnastics, diving, high jump, pentathlon and soccer in the case of people with learning disabilities and cervical spine instability, particularly those with Down syndrome and atlanto-axial instability. However, restricting the involvement in sporting activities of people with learning disabilities remains controversial.

Disorders of vision

Ocular abnormalities are common in people with learning disabilities, with virtually all structures of the eye having been reported to have some associated abnormality. Visual impairment involves a loss in visual acuity, resulting in partial sight to total blindness. Impairment is 10 to 15 times greater in people with severe learning disabilities compared with the general population. The prevalence increases with age (1 in 3 elderly people may have some impairment present), myopia, hypermetropia and astigmatism being common causes of visual impair-ment. It is usually possible to test vision with standard charts, but the presence of nystagmus and poor co-operation may make assessment of visual acuity difficult.

A number of specific ophthalmic abnormalities are associated with specific syndromes (e.g. cataracts with Down syndrome and optic atrophy with cerebral palsy). Impairment of vision in a person with learning disabilities can lead to difficulties in communication, loss of mobility and a general decline in social skills.

Blepharitis is common, but is usually amenable to daily washing with water and/or baby shampoo. Severe infections may require antibiotics. Keratoconus (conical cornea) is a disorder of the cornea of the eye and is particularly associated with Down syndrome. Cataracts are also associated with increasing age in adults with Down syndrome (the prevalence ranges from 25% to 85%). Blindness can result if there is no surgical intervention. However, only a small percentage of affected individuals undergo surgical intervention. The aetiology remains unknown.

Other common abnormalities of the eye include strabismus, nystagmus and less common retina anomalies (e.g. an increased number of retinal blood vessels crossing the disc margin), retinoblastoma, amblyopia (unilateral decreased visual acuity) and ectropions.

The majority of people with learning disabilities have some abnormality of the eye, but very few of these individuals ever receive appropriate care. The possibility of visual problems should always be considered when a person with learning disabilities begins to lose interest in daily living skills. Many of the pathologies are treatable, and early detection and management can prevent future visual loss and continue to maintain the individual's quality of life. For people who already have one handicap, prevention of another is of paramount importance. Improved screening, provision of spectacles and magnifying glasses, and increased awareness of the problem among professionals and carers can reduce the effects of this dual disability. Changes in the environment (e.g. use of contrasting colours, provision of guide rails, adapting light levels and provision of easier-to-use objects) can also improve the quality of life.

Hearing

Hearing problems are also more common in people with learning disabilities (Van Schrojenstein Lantman-de Valk *et al.* 2000). Prevalence rates for hearing impairment range from 6.8% to 56.7% (Yeates 1992; Evenhuis *et al.* 2001), with rates being significantly higher for older people and for individuals with Down syndrome.

Types of hearing loss include sensorineural deafness (30%), conductive deafness (10%), mixed (28%) and unknown (30%). The normal range of hearing is for sounds of between 0 and 15 decibels in frequency. There is a slight loss of hearing when the intensity of sound has to be between 15 and 25 decibels, mild loss at 25 to 40 decibels, moderate loss at 40 to 65 decibels, severe loss at 65 to 95 decibels and profound loss at 95 decibels or more.

Conductive loss can be due to the presence of wax or middle ear effusions, and sensorineural hearing loss can be due to impairment in nerve conduction. Conductive loss is more common. Sensorineural loss is probably related to accelerated ageing, but possibly also to chronic middle ear disease affecting neural structures.

Several researchers have demonstrated that individuals with impaired hearing have impaired social functioning (Wright *et al.* 1991), and that hearing loss may be a factor in decline in cognitive functioning and in auditory–verbal processing.

If hearing loss is suspected, hearing tests should be performed by an audiologist with experience of working with people with learning disabilities. Auditory brainstem responses may be used if standard audiometry proves difficult to perform (Evenhuis *et al.* 1992). Removal of wax may lead to immediate benefit, but the removal of chronic impacted wax is less likely to improve hearing. Middle ear effusions may require surgical intervention with the insertion of grommets. The response to the use of a hearing aid can be excellent, although many people with learning disabilities may initially refuse to wear them. However, with ongoing support and training of the individual and carers, hearing aids can be successfully used.

Infections can be up to 100 times more common in people with learning disabilities, and infections of the nose and throat may lead to involvement of the middle ear. The cause of the increased susceptibility to infections is unknown, but may be associated with a depressed immune system, anatomical abnormalities and poor oral hygiene.

People with learning disabilities should be screened regularly for hearing problems. Chronic recurrent infections may be treated with long-term antibiotics, but surgical intervention may be necessary for middle ear effusions. Frequent cleaning will help to prevent wax impaction. Any resulting hearing loss may be improved by the use of hearing aids.

Oral health

People with learning disabilities are predisposed to the following:

1   oral ill health, due to dental factors such as reduced flow of saliva making plaque deposits dense and sticky
2   peridontal and gingival ill health, due to a tendency to mouth breathe, which makes the lips and tongue dry
3   impaired control and movement of the tongue, making the removal of food from the mouth more difficult
4   poor manual dexterity, which may pose problems in brushing the teeth properly
5   malocclusions.

In addition, complicating factors such as side-effects of treatment (e.g. thickening of the gums with phenytoin), behavioural difficulties and the presence of medical factors such as specific syndromes lead to dental and peridontal disease.

People with learning disabilities have a high prevalence of malocclusions. These include lower facial anomalies and cross-biting. There is an increased prevalence of dental anomalies (e.g. absent teeth, peg-shaped incisors, microdontia, loss of alveolar bone). Periodontal disease, including necrotising ulcerative gingivitis, is very common, and its prevalence increases with age.

Aetiological factors are probably multi-factorial, but anatomical abnormalities, saliva changes and differences in vascular supply to the lower half of the head may predispose to pathology. Abnormalities of the immune system probably play an important role. Residents in institutions also appear to be at greater risk of periodontal disease.

Several recommendations for improving the oral hygiene of people with learning disabilities can be made, including the following:

1   regular dental assessments with a focus on prevention
2   increasing carers' awareness of the importance of oral hygiene
3   oral hygiene may be supplemented with chemical and antibacterial plaque control (e.g. chlorhexidine)
4   giving advice on a suitable type of toothbrush, including individual adaptations and the correct method of brushing the teeth
5   dietary advice
6   the importance of topical fluoride application where appropriate
7   the use of sugar-free medication.

Skin disorders

Skin complaints that occur in the general population may also occur in people with learning disabilities. However, particular problems are dry skin, atopic dermatitis, alopecia areata, psoriasis and tinea pedis. Dry skin can occur in up to 70–85% of individuals with Down syndrome (Carter and Jegasothy 1976), and is best managed by using oil-based soaps, keeping the skin hydrated, and using moisturisers and emollients. Atopic dermatitis can occur at any age, and may be treated by using non-perfumed soaps and bath oils and improving hydration of the skin. Antihistamines and steroid creams can be helpful.

Seborrhoeic dermatitis and alopecia areata (loss of hair) occur less commonly, may involve the scalp hair, beard and eyelashes, and can be quite severe. The aetiology of hair loss is unknown, but it is probably autoimmune and genetic in origin. Treatable causes such as hypothyroidism (Scotson 1989) and adrenal failure (Bergfield 1988) have to be ruled out. Complete regrowth can occur spontaneously, although numerous treatment regimes using allopathic agents (e.g. steroids) and alternative therapies have been used with minimal effect (Burke 1989).

Skin complaints are common in people with learning disabilities. Irritation and considerable distress can result, leading to behavioural difficulties. Simple effective measures have been shown to be beneficial.

Endocrine disorders

Normal endocrine function is dependent on a number of organ systems within the human body. Normal functioning of the hypothalamus and pituitary gland in the brain is central to maintaining normal hormonal levels. Important organs that are involved include the thyroid gland, pancreas and adrenal glands.

The most widely researched endocrine disorder in the context of learning disabilities is thyroid dysfunction in people with Down syndrome. Such an association has now been well established, with underactivity (hypothyroidism) and overactivity (hyperthyroidism) due to congenital and acquired causes being more common than in the general population. The prevalence of thyroid dysfunction increases with age, with up to 50% of adults with Down syndrome over the age of 40 years showing some evidence of thyroid dysfunction. An association between thyroid autoimmunity and thyroid dysfunction has been reported.

It may be difficult to diagnose hypothyroidism clinically, as some of the features (e.g. lethargy and weight gain) may already be present (Prasher 1995). Regular biochemical screening for thyroid dysfunction is therefore recommended. The current guidelines are that individuals with previously normal thyroid function should be tested every 2 years, while those with a history of thyroid disease should be tested annually.

Treatment of hypothyroidism has been shown to be beneficial, and a number of case reports have been published in which, for example, alopecia totalis or total hair loss has been reversed, pseudodementia has resolved and an increase in social functioning has been achieved after the administration of thyroxine replacement therapy.

Other disorders associated with hypothyroidism in people with Down syndrome include hypoparathyroidism, diabetes mellitus and precocious sexual development. A possible association between Alzheimer's disease and thyroid dysfunction in adults with Down syndrome remains an interesting area for future research.

Primary healthcare models

People with learning disabilities are susceptible to many physical illnesses, which affect virtually all organs and bodily systems. The prevalence of such disorders is higher than that for the general population, and can have a considerable impact on the life of a person with learning disabilities. Significant emotional and/or behavioural disturbance and loss of adaptive skills may result.

With growing numbers of adults with learning disabilities surviving to middle age and beyond, it is essential that medical care keeps pace. Deficiencies in healthcare provision may lead to physical illnesses being missed and to mis-diagnosis of both medical and psychiatric conditions. In order to achieve and maintain a high quality of life for people with learning disabilities, care professionals must be aware of the associated illnesses. Furthermore, many people with learning disabilities may be unable to verbalise the presence of pain, carers may not seek help and staff may be unaware of the presence of associated physical disorders. People with learning disabilities thus have difficulties in accessing health services, in particular screening, dental and primary healthcare services. As a result, significant physical morbidity may remain inadequately treated.

Martin and Roy (1999) have reviewed the models of primary healthcare that have been used so far. They include the general practitioner-led approach, the specialist-led approach and collaborative models.

General practitioner-led approach

As the title suggests, in this model the general practitioners have taken the lead in initiating health screening. Howells (1986) offered health checks to people with learning disabilities attending a training centre, and found a significant number of unmanaged physical disorders.

Kerr et al. (1996) conducted a comprehensive health check for 28 people with learning disabilities and compared them with matched controls in a practice-based study. It was found that the study group received less of the regular screening (i.e. immunisation and cervical cytology) but had more outpatient appointments and saw more specialists.

Specialist-led approach

In this model, the specialist, usually the consultant psychiatrist, has taken the lead in conducting health checks. A study by Wilson and Haire (1990) of people with learning disabilities attending an adult training centre in Nottingham is an example of this model. Beange et al. (1995) conducted a community-based study in the Northshore district of Sydney, Australia. As in other studies, a higher incidence of unmanaged health problems was demonstrated in both cases.

Collaborative models

This approach involves collaboration between the primary healthcare team and the specialist services in providing comprehensive health checks. In the first of these models, a facilitator coordinated people with learning disabilities having a health check at their own general practitioner's surgery (Martin *et al.* 1997). Bollard (1998) has discussed a model in which the Community Learning Disability Nurse's role was extended to work with the primary healthcare team. Health checks offered at GP practices were performed mainly by practice nurses. Cassidy *et al.* (2002) have described joint clinics for people with learning disabilities where physical and psychiatric health checks are offered during a single visit to the surgery.

In order to reduce the number of undetected health problems of people with learning disabilities, further training is needed for medical students and general practitioners. Plant (1997) demonstrated by means of a confidential postal questionnaire that general practitioners often lacked confidence in caring for people with learning disabilities. There is some confusion about what constitutes a learning disability, the different degrees of learning disability, the health needs that people with learning disabilities have and the configuration of specialist services, although general practitioners are often in the position of knowing a great deal about these individuals' social situations (Marshall *et al.* 1996). This can lead to practices rejecting people with learning disabilities because of the 'perceived increase in workload' (Chambers 1998). Chambers argues for general practitioners to be given 'protected paid time' in which to carry out proactive work. Equally, financial incentives can improve patient compliance (Giuffrida and Torgerson 1997).

The importance of primary healthcare in the general population has been recognised by successive governments. The *Health of the Nation* objectives for people with learning disabilities focused on improvement of both their physical and mental health. The White Paper entitled *The New NHS: modern, dependable* (Department of Health 1997) acknowledges the role of primary healthcare. The concepts within that document (e.g. the establishment of primary care groups and clinical governance at primary care level) represent opportunities to improve and maintain the health of this vulnerable group. Improvement in the arena of physical health will eventually improve their quality of life. Guidance has been published on health facilitation and health action plans as a means of improving the health of people with learning disabilities (Department of Health 2002) by adopting the twin approach of accessing family doctors and adopting healthier lifestyles (*see* Chapter 14).

References

Beange H, McElduff A and Baker W (1995) Medical disorders of adults with mental retardation: a population study. *Am J Ment Retard.* 99: 595–604.

Bergfield WF (1988) Etiology and diagnosis of androgenic alopecia. *Clin Dermatol.* 6: 102–7.

Bollard M (1998) *Collaboration with the PHCT: findings from a pilot project within GP practices.* Private communication.

Braun DL, Green MD, Rausen AR *et al.* (1985) Down's syndrome and testicular cancer: a possible association. *J Pediatr Hematol Oncol.* 7: 208–11.

Burke KE (1989) Hair loss: what causes it and what can be done about it. *Postgrad Med.* **85:** 67–77.

Carter DM and Jegasothy BV (1976) Alopecia areata and Down syndrome. *Arch Dermatol.* **112:** 1397–9.

Cassidy G, Martin DM, Martin GHB and Roy A (2002) Health checks for people with learning disabilities: community learning disability teams working together with general practitioners and primary health care teams. *J Learn Disabil.* **6**(2): 123–36.

Chambers R (1998) The primary care workload and prescribing costs associated with patients with learning disability discharged from long-stay care to the community. *Br J Learn Disabil.* **26:** 9–12.

Cohen J (2001) Countries' health performance. *Lancet.* **358:** 929.

Department of Health (1995) *The Health of a Nation. A strategy for people with learning disabilities.* HMSO, London.

Department of Health (1997) *The New NHS: modern, dependable.* Department of Health, London.

Department of Health (2002) *Action for Health: health action plans and health facilitation detailed good practice guidance on implementation for learning disability partnership boards.* Department of Health, London.

Evenhuis HM, van Zanten GA, Brocaar MP and Roerdinkholder WHM (1992) Hearing loss in middle-aged persons with Down syndrome. *Am J Ment Retard.* **97:** 47–56.

Evenhuis HM, Theunissen M, Denkers I, Verschuure H and Kemme H (2001) Prevalence of visual and hearing impairment in a Dutch institutionalized population with intellectual disability. *J Intellect Defic Res.* **45:** 457–64.

Giuffrida A and Torgerson DT (1997) Should we pay the patient? Review of financial incentives to enhance patient compliance. *BMJ.* **315:** 703–7.

Howells G (1986) Are the health care needs of mentally handicapped adults being met? *J R Coll Gen Pract.* **36:** 449–53.

Kerr MP, Richards D and Glover G (1996) Primary care for people with an intellectual disability: a group practice survey. *J Appl Res Intellect Disabil.* **9:** 347–52.

Marshall S, Martin DM and Myles F (1996) Survey of GPs' views of learning disabilities services. *Br J Nurs.* **5:** 488–93.

Martin DM, Roy A and Wells MB (1997) Health gains through health checks: improving access to primary health care for people with intellectual disability. *J Intellect Disabil Res.* **41:** 401–8.

Martin D and Roy A (1999) A comparative review of primary health care models for people with learning disabilities: towards the provision of seamless health care. *Br J Learn Disabil.* **27:** 58–63.

Moss S, Goldberg D, Patel P and Wilkin D (1993) Physical morbidity in people with moderate, severe and profound mental handicap, and its relation to psychiatric morbidity. *Soc Psychiatry Psychiatr Epidemiol.* **28:** 32–9.

Plant M (1997) The provision of primary health care for adults who have learning disabilities. *Br J Dev Disabil.* **43:** 75–8.

Prasher VP (1994) Screening of physical morbidity in adults with Down syndrome. *Down Syndrome Res Pract.* **2:** 59–66.

Prasher VP (1995) Overweight and obesity amongst Down syndrome adults. *J Intellect Disabil Res.* **39:** 437–41.

Richards BW and Enver F (1979) Blood pressure in Down's syndrome. *J Ment Defic Res.* **23:** 123–35.

Scotson J (1989) A patient with Down's syndrome, mild hypothyroidism and alopecia. *Practitioner.* **233:** 121.

Stewart L, Beange H and McKerras D (1994) A survey of dietary problems of adults with learning disabilities in the community. *Ment Handicap Res.* **7:** 41–50.

Van Schrojenstein Lantman-de Valk HMJ, Metsemakers JFM, Haveman MJ and Crebolder

HFJM (2000) Health problems in people with intellectual disability in general practice: a comparative study. *Fam Pract.* **17:** 405–7.

Wilson DN and Haire A (1990) Health care screening for people with mental handicap living in the community. *BMJ.* **301:** 1379–81.

Wingfield M, Healy DL and Nicholson A (1994) Gynaecological care for women with intellectual disability. *Med J Aust.* **160:** 536–8.

Wright PF, Thompson J and Bess FH (1991) Hearing, speech and language sequelae of otitis media with effusion. *Pediatr Ann.* **20:** 617–21.

Yeates S (1992) Have they got a hearing loss? A follow-up study of hearing in people with mental handicap. *Mental Handicap.* **20:** 126–33.

Chapter 8

Psychiatric and behaviour disorders in children and adolescents with intellectual disabilities

Pru Allington-Smith

Introduction

Young people with a learning disability are not a homogenous group. They vary in their level of cognitive impairment, whether they have an autistic spectrum disorder or not, the presence of other disabilities, the cause of the impairment, their families and, last but by no means least, their personalities. Each is a unique individual who comes from a distinct family.

Population studies show that children and adolescents with a learning disability have a much higher incidence of psychiatric illness and challenging behaviour. The Isle of Wight study conducted by Michael Rutter (1976) and his colleagues looked at all of the children aged 10–12 years on the island in order to identify those who had a psychiatric disorder. Greatly increased rates of psychiatric disorder were found in children who had a global intellectual disability, epilepsy or cerebral palsy. A later study showed the same increase in children who suffered from brain damage following an accident. Where one or more of these conditions was present the risks were cumulative. John Corbett (1979), in his Camberwell study, found an overall rate of 47% for psychiatric and behavioural disorders in children with a severe or profound learning disability. Similarly high figures were reported by Gillberg *et al.* (1986).

Although precise data are difficult to obtain, the British Paediatric Association (1994) estimated that an average district with a population of 250 000 would be expected to have 200 children with a severe learning disability. In their study of challenging behaviour, Kiernan and Quereshi (1993) estimated that in this population there would be approximately 25 children whose severe learning disability was associated with challenging behaviours that posed a serious management problem.

Due to the nature and complexity of these children, they are best managed by a multi-disciplinary approach drawing on the appropriate resources from education, social services and healthcare. Each professional needs to work not only with the young person but also with their family, and liaison with colleagues from other disciplines is essential. Listening to parents provides the main source of information, and workers ignore the parents' insights at their peril. Harsh judgements are sometimes made about the family's coping strategy, but the professional must imagine how they would cope given the family set-up and circumstances. Imposing ideas without engaging the family will seldom lead to any improvement in the life of the young person.

Services

The services available to these young people vary widely according to geographical location in the UK. A child with a behavioural or psychiatric problem may be referred to learning disability psychiatrists, child psychiatrists or clinical psychologists, often depending on which professional has a special interest and the requisite skills. In a few areas none of these professionals are willing or able to see these children, and their care may be left to learning disability nurses, paediatricians or community paediatricians, who often lack the skills to manage major behavioural or psychiatric disorders. Examples of specialist coordinated services do exist. For the child with a behavioural or psychiatric problem, the core team would ideally include community learning disability nurses, clinical psychologists, a learning disability and/or child psychiatrist, communication (speech and language) therapists, occupational therapists and a dietitian. These team members would work closely with community paediatricians, teachers, school nurses, educational psychologists and social workers. Other professionals may also have an important role.

Assessment

A full assessment starts with a comprehensive history of the child and their family. It may be possible to interview the young person on their own, as well as the parents. Additional information should be sought (with parental permission) from the school, community nurses, respite workers and other professionals who have been involved with the child. A visit to the school is often illuminating. It is often easier to take the initial history from the parents at the school, and to see the child afterwards. Children with severe behavioural problems may present very differently in environments other than home. It is also helpful to make at least one home visit.

Particular emphasis should be placed on the duration and frequency of the presenting problems and any precipitating factors. It is important to assess the level of learning disability, although a formal psychometric assessment (IQ test) is seldom necessary within a health setting, except where there is a marked disparity between the child's various abilities. It is important to establish how well the child or young person is able to communicate his or her wishes. It is vital to document the presence or absence of an autistic spectrum disorder, as this has profound implications not only for how the child should be taught but also for the management of the presenting problem. Traditional behavioural approaches do not always work with a child who has an autistic spectrum disorder, and they sometimes make things worse. In addition to giving specific advice on how to manage behaviours, it is vital that the parents and teachers have a good understanding of what autism is, so that they can begin to understand what the child's perception of his or her world is likely to be.

If possible, it is important to identify the aetiology of the learning disability. Some genetic conditions are associated with physical disorders that may need treatment or ongoing monitoring (e.g. tuberous sclerosis). Most of these investigations are undertaken by paediatricians in the first three years of the child's life, but they may not have been done, particularly if the child presents later. It is still not possible to make a definitive diagnosis in up to 50% of all children with a learning disability. Some genetic conditions may be associated with particular patterns of behaviour, the so-called *behavioural phenotype*, and knowledge of these can be very helpful in management. Examples of recognised behavioural phenotypes include fragile X syndrome, Prader–Willi syndrome and Lesch–Nyhan syndrome.

A full medical history should be sought as many children, especially those with a severe or profound impairment, have multiple disabilities. It is particularly important to ask about visual and hearing impairments. The child should be examined and, if necessary, investigations should be ordered. Physical illness should always be eliminated as a cause of behavioural problems, particularly if the behaviour is of relatively recent onset. Chronic dental or ear infections will lead to distress and perhaps head banging. Orthopaedic problems are common (e.g. dislocated hips in a child who sits in a wheelchair all day). Some parents are not aware that some of the conditions can be alleviated, and it is sometimes necessary to ask colleagues for procedures that would automatically be offered to 'normal' children.

Epilepsy is particularly common in this group and may not have been recognised, particularly if the child has absence seizures. Epilepsy can have a profound impact on the child's behaviour even if there are few overt seizures. Where any doubt exists it is worth obtaining an electroencephalogram (EEG). The treatment of epilepsy may cause its own problems. Some drugs can affect behaviour and even occasionally provoke a serious psychiatric illness (*see* Chapter 7). Many side-effects are very predictable, such as drowsiness or mental slowing, and are likely to be noticed by the parents. Other common side-effects, such as blurred vision, may go unrecognised because the child cannot or does not complain. It is therefore important to report any unusual behaviours. Some drugs, most notably carbamazepine and phenytoin, can be monitored by means of blood tests and the dosage adjusted accordingly. Newer anti-epileptic drugs have become available in recent years, some of which have specific problems associated with them. Some of these drugs (e.g. vigabatrin, which can cause peripheral visual loss) are best avoided in children who cannot be adequately tested or monitored.

Common disorders in children with learning disabilities

Temper tantrums

A child who is developing normally will frequently display extreme reactions to being denied what they want. The 'terrible twos' are aptly named. As the child's reasoning abilities develop, so does their capacity to wait for what they want or to cope with disappointment. A child with learning disabilities may not achieve this level of reasoning until much later, if at all, and so may continue to behave in a similar way to a normal 2-year-old, but with more destructive and frightening consequences, as they get bigger and stronger. Less than ideal management of a normal 2-year-old does not matter too much, as the child will eventually grow out of the habit, but for parents of a child with learning disabilities inappropriate management can lead to major difficulties if it is not corrected early on.

Parents realise that to give in to the child's demands during a temper tantrum is not the right thing to do, but often weaken their resolve in the face of continuing shouting, screaming, destruction and/or physical aggression directed towards a sibling, the parents or expressed as self-injury. The sad fact is that the behaviours will continue if there remains the smallest chance that the child will get what they want. It is only if the parents are completely consistent in 'saying no and meaning it' that the behaviours are likely to stop. Parents have to be taught to give attention to the child when he or she is acting appropriately and not when the child is misbehaving. In the short term, when parents begin to take this firm line, the situation will even get worse as the child tries to find the parents' breaking point. If this can be endured, the eventual results are more than worth the struggle. This is obviously easier to achieve with a young or physically small child. Some parents express the idea that because the child has disabilities, they have the right to have whatever they want when they want, as if this will somehow make up for their life difficulties. However, no one wins with temper tantrums, as the child does not enjoy the behaviour and has no idea how to bring it to an end.

General behavioural guidelines can be helpful for parents, and include the following:

- ignoring unwanted behaviours whenever possible
- persistently praising desired behaviour
- when intervention is needed, remaining calm and not shouting
- both parents agreeing on the approach to be taken to unwanted behaviours, and working together
- not threatening the child with withdrawing something that they know will happen anyway (e.g. 'no Christmas presents')
- when saying no, sticking to their intentions
- only giving a single warning to the child that if they do not comply there will be consequences.

On some occasions a period of 'time out' can be helpful. In this case it is briefly explained to the child what they have done wrong. The child is then led to a quiet and boring area of the house where they must remain for a short time (the time will vary from 3 to 10 minutes depending on the age and understanding of the child, but once chosen should remain the same). The parent must remain calm at all times and not talk to the child once they are in time out. The child is free to return after the allotted time and should not be chastised further. If the behaviour is repeated and a single warning is ignored, the child should be returned to repeat 'time out'. At first this may have to take place several times before the child realises the consequences of their undesired actions. Later in the day, when the situation is fully over, the parent may discuss with the child in a calm and positive manner what the correct behaviour should have been.

Most children thrive on attention, and although they prefer it to be positive, will settle for criticism or even physical chastisement if nothing else is forthcoming. It is therefore vital to spend time encouraging the child in desirable activities and not leaving them alone because, for once, they are being quiet. A child can only model their behaviour on what is going on around them. If the child hears the parent shouting and swearing, then that is what they will do too, only louder!

For a child with an autistic spectrum disorder, the above often does not apply. Tantrums in an autistic child are frequently a response to overwhelming anxiety. These children find it very difficult to cope with new situations and people, as they see them as unpredictable and therefore potentially threatening. Becoming very upset in these situations will usually result in the 'threat' being removed or the child being taken back to a familiar environment. If they are then told off, this is incomprehensible to the child and may increase the level of distress. Preparing the child before they encounter a new situation can often reduce the frequency of such episodes. This preparation may be done verbally, but it is often best to reinforce it with visual cues such as symbols, photographs or objects of reference (e.g. a seat-belt buckle to represent a car journey).

Children with autistic disorders (see also *Chapter 4*)

The diagnosis of autistic spectrum disorders in children is one of the main reasons for referral to psychiatric services. A diagnosis can be made reliably in children as young as 18 months, depending on the severity of the autism and the presence of any other disabilities. The more severe the degree of learning disability, the greater the prevalence of an autistic disorder. In children with a severe or profound learning disability (IQ below 30), a diagnosis of atypical autism is most likely. This does not imply that these children are less autistic, but rather that they do not have enough abilities, either intellectually or physically, to demonstrate the full range of autistic traits. Children with an autistic spectrum disorder and a learning disability are much more likely to develop serious behavioural problems than children who just have a learning disability. They represent nearly all those with seriously challenging behaviours, such as aggression to others or self-injury. These young people are often chronically anxious, and it can take very little to provoke them into a state where they lose control. The behaviours are most often directed towards parents and siblings. It is not at all uncommon for an autistic child to behave well at school, trying desperately to conform, only to erupt in fury at the day's events the moment they walk through their own front door. The basis for management is to maximise the child's communication and understanding and to improve their physical environment. Giving the child a certain amount of predictability to their day and a calm place in which to unwind when they are upset can also be of benefit. If these measures have been employed and the behaviours still persist and are clearly linked to anxiety, there may be a case for using medication. These medications include selective serotonin reuptake inhibitors (e.g. fluoxetine), carbamazepine or very-low-dose risperidone. None of these medications are licensed for use in autism, and they should only be prescribed by a specialist after a careful evaluation.

Recognition of the condition has important implications for educational provision for the child, and it may influence which school the child attends or the method of teaching that is employed in the classroom. Increasingly, preschool interventions such as 'Early Bird' are being offered to the parents and child after the initial diagnosis has been made. With more children now being diagnosed, greater demands for specialist autism educational provision have come from parents. Most areas are now responding to these demands, although relatively few areas have adequate resources at present. In the case of children who also have a learning disability, each needs to be assessed individually when choosing the most suitable school for them. Some will do better in schools for children with autism, while others will flourish in 'ordinary' special schools, most of which now employ specific teaching methods for this group of children or contain autism units. Services for adults with a learning disability have so far largely failed to respond to the growing need for specific provision.

Time spent educating parents about the condition gives them a better insight into the way that their child perceives his or her world. This in turn leads to more effective behavioural management at home, as well as increased empathy with the child. Parents have often been told that their child is just naughty or that they are failing as parents. The child's behaviour is usually bizarre and sometimes frightening. At the time of referral, parents are often demoralised and experiencing feelings of guilt or blame. To finally be given an explanation as to why their child behaves as he or she does nearly always comes as an enormous relief. Families can be given contact details for the various autism family support organisations, most of which are excellent.

Sleep disorders

Sleep problems are one of the parents' main complaints. In extreme cases they can result in the child having to move away from home because of parental exhaustion. Many children with a severe learning disability, especially those who also have an autistic spectrum disorder, seem to have a decreased need for sleep. The child may not settle in bed at night, or may wake frequently or early. Poor sleep is sometimes associated with daytime drowsiness and irritability in the child. Establishing a good bedtime routine and a firm approach to the management of waking can help some families. It is surprising how many parents admit that their child has a television, DVD player and computer games in his or her bedroom. In other cases, behavioural techniques may be ineffective. Medication has a limited role in management. Virtually all of the available preparations affect the child during the day to some extent, and drug tolerance quickly develops. These 'hypnotic' medications may have a useful role if used intermittently, when tolerance does not usually occur. For children with a severe learning disability or autism, melatonin can be helpful. This is a synthetic version of a naturally occurring hormone that is secreted by the pineal gland in the brain. Its secretion is increased before the onset of sleep and during the night, and is influenced by the level of light outside. By giving the hormone before the desired bedtime, induction of sleep may be achieved. It is less effective in children who wake during the night. The hormone appears to be relatively safe and has antioxidant properties. It seems to have a variable effect on epilepsy, improving control in some cases but worsening it in others (Coppola *et al.* 2004).

Attention deficit hyperactivity disorder (ADHD)

This disorder is characterised by marked over-activity, inattention and poor impulse control that is inappropriate for the child's developmental level. It is common in children with a learning disability, but can be difficult to diagnose accurately. The triad of symptoms may also be present in children with poorly controlled epilepsy and in those with autism. Symptoms should be present in more than one environment (i.e. at home and at school). The child will have demonstrated these problems from an early age, and often sleeps poorly. ADHD may respond to behavioural management, and usually responds to medication. The first line of drug treatment is still stimulant medications such as methylphenidate. The non-stimulant atomoxetine has recently become available in the UK. Medication should only be used after careful assessment and with close supervision. If it is effective, treatment may need to continue for several years, and during that time growth and blood pressure should be checked regularly. Children with a learning disability seem to be more prone to the side-effects associated with stimulant use, especially a reduction in appetite.

Depression

Adolescents are most likely to suffer this disorder, although it is by no means unknown in younger children. It is characterised by low mood that is present for the majority of the time and which has been present for more than 3 weeks. The child may be weepy, withdrawn and disinterested. Sleep, appetite and concentration may be impaired in more severe cases. In children with a more severe learning disability the presentation may be different, with an increase in stereotypical behaviour (e.g. rocking, self-injury) and irritability. There are many causes of depression, and episodes may resolve when the cause is removed or the child is able in some way to express how they feel. Some children have a strong family history of the condition, and episodes may have no discernible cause. Most treatments are psychological, although the most severely affected children may benefit from antidepressant medication. The cognitive behavioural techniques that have been employed so successfully in mainstream child psychiatry are not easily adaptable to learning-disabled children. Teenagers with a mild learning disability are particularly vulnerable to feelings of depression when they begin to appreciate that they are different from other children and more dependent on their parents. Complete social withdrawal may occur in young people with autism who feel that the world is too difficult and threatening for them to be in it. They may refuse to go to school and can become housebound.

Eating problems

Poor appetite and poor weight gain are common in young children who have a learning disability. Tube or gastrostomy feeding may become necessary in a few children with a profound disability. This type of feeding is sometimes associated with reflux of the stomach contents back up the oesophagus, causing irritation and ulceration. In milder cases this can usually be controlled with medication, but if severe it may require surgery. Reflux can also occur in a child with no physical disabilities, particularly if they have autism, and may be related to the way in which the child chews and swallows. A speech and language therapist's assessment of and advice on chewing and swallowing can be invaluable.

Feeding difficulties in a child with autism may arise because of refusal to try new foods, or because the child dislikes certain food textures or smells. Most children when hungry enough will overcome their dislikes, but the autistic child may well prefer to starve. Anorexia nervosa (causing severe weight loss because of food refusal and fear of fatness) is uncommon.

Overeating is more common in older children, and can be a source of considerable conflict between the parent and child. In children with Prader–Willi syndrome (*see* Chapter 6), overeating can result in life-threatening obesity, although as infants these children have feeding problems. At some point between 1 and 3 years of age, the child's appetite increases markedly and, unless the parents are told what could happen, gains huge amounts of weight rapidly. These children are prone to temper tantrums, often over demands for food. Many parents have to resort to locking kitchen cupboards and the fridge.

Whether a child is over- or underweight, it is inadvisable to use food as a reward for desired behaviour, not least because the foods that the child most values often have the least nutritional value.

Childhood neurosis

Anxiety in children is common, and may range from a simple dog or spider phobia to a severe separation anxiety that prevents the child from attending school. Constantly high anxiety levels are nearly always present in children with autism, and arise from a fear of new situations or people. Obsessional behaviour is nearly always present in autism, but can be present in other children as part of an obsessive-compulsive disorder. Some children with learning disabilities demonstrate lesser degrees of this behaviour, with excessive tidiness and an unwillingness to try new things. This could be interpreted as an attempt to impose structure and order in a world over which they have little influence. Most neurotic conditions in children who do not have autism respond well to behavioural therapies, and medication is seldom indicated. Occasionally medication can be helpful in children with autistic spectrum disorders.

Family factors

Every family has its own strengths and weaknesses. Having a child with a learning disability will inevitably challenge a family's resources. Many cope very well and find the experience a totally positive one. Of course some children are much more difficult to deal with than others, being emotionally unresponsive, overactive or physically unattractive. Parents may be unsupported, socially isolated and have marital difficulties. Single parents and those families where one or both parents have had to give up work in order to become full-time carers may have low incomes. Parents may have unresolved issues concerning having given birth to a 'handicapped' child. They may continue to mourn for the child they expected to have, or search tirelessly for a diagnosis or 'cure', refusing to accept the extent of their child's problem. Some parents may themselves have a significant learning disability. Support from members of a community learning disability team is usually available, and respite care, sitting services or shared care with another family are often accessible, although in short supply. Family therapy to discuss parent–child problems can be invaluable.

Adolescence

As we grow older we acquire physical and mental skills. We do this partly by exploring our physical environment and by being allowed to take risks. It is also by learning to disagree with parents and teachers that we develop a sense of our own identity. For a young adult with a learning disability, adolescence often occurs late and is prolonged. Leaving school, instead of bringing greater independence, can lead to the opposite situation.

Parents of young people with learning disabilities often need to provide more care and more guidance for their children. It is extremely hard to allow a child to do something on their own in the knowledge that they are likely to fail – not once but repeatedly. If the child has an additional problem (e.g. poor vision or epilepsy), it is even harder. Therefore it is not surprising that many parents are overprotective – not allowing their child to risk failure, and thereby denying them opportunities to learn and to gain some independence. Children are encouraged to be as independent as possible at school, and then become very frustrated by the restrictions imposed on them at home. The young adult may seek an area of control in the household, and may use his or her strength in order to get it. By working with the whole family, these issues can be explored and resolved.

School-related problems

For parents, one of the hardest times is the assessment period prior to their child starting school. They are often uncertain whether the child would do best in a special school or in a supported mainstream placement. The trend at present is for educational psychologists to recommend that if at all possible the child should start out in the local school. This has obvious advantages, as they will not have to travel far and they will meet neighbouring children and have the opportunity to form friendships. They will then have these children as a role model for behaviour.

Some children will be unable to manage in mainstream schools even with considerable support. The school may lack the skills necessary to manage behavioural problems or to present work to the child at the appropriate level. As the child grows older, the difference between them and their classmates becomes more pronounced. The child may be teased or bullied, and will often start to realise that they cannot work as successfully as those around them. This may lead to reluctance to undertake tasks, so that they do not have to demonstrate their deficiencies. In older children, school refusal may be the ultimate result. Children are continually assessed throughout school, and in some areas they are transferred to special schools if necessary. This service may be delayed or unavailable in those areas where special schools have been phased out. The child is sometimes left with the feeling that they have failed. Indeed, lack of self-esteem is a feature that all of these children have in common, even in the best environments. It is vital that the child is placed where they can succeed at their level, and that they are not given work that is beyond their capabilities. It is also essential that schools have the ability to cope with the very significant number of children whose behaviour causes problems.

Sexual and physical abuse

Only in recent times has the sexual abuse of children been acknowledged by society. Recognition of the problem in the learning disabled has taken even longer, and has been termed 'thinking the unthinkable'. The sad fact is that children with learning disabilities are more vulnerable than 'normal' children. They may be unable to communicate distress effectively, and are easily intimidated. Many abused children who could talk reported that they felt no one would believe them or that if bad things happened to them they somehow deserved it. Children with learning disabilities may have multiple carers, and this increases the risk of coming into contact with an abuser although 50% of all abuse takes place within the family. All health, education and social workers who come into contact with children will have a police check, and it is vital that private and voluntary organisations submit their staff to the same procedures. Parents unfortunately need to maintain a high degree of suspicion if the child's behaviour deteriorates after they have been in a specific setting. Help is available for children who have been sexually, physically or emotionally abused, although the work needed is often long-term, and permanent emotional damage is common.

Young people who offend

The vast majority of learning-disabled offenders have a mild impairment. These young people are easily led by other children into petty crime, as a result of which they are nearly always caught because of their lack of sophistication. Arson and sexual offences are the most frequently encountered serious offences. Treatment programmes are being developed for adults with a learning disability who offend, and the principles that these programmes utilise can be employed with children. In the case of arsonists, the main aim is for the offender to realise the potential risk to others of what they are doing. Sexual offenders have often been abused themselves or are seeking out sexual partners of a similar developmental level to themselves. Their treatment usually involves sex education, the development of empathy for their victims, and often work on the abuse to which they have been subjected in the past.

Outlook

The emotional needs of children and adolescents who have a learning disability are now being recognised, and specific services are being developed to help them and their families. Many factors are often involved, and help can be drawn from sources in health, education, social services and the voluntary and private sector. These efforts need to be coordinated and advertised so that families know what is available. The aim is for children to grow up emotionally stable so that they can use what abilities they have to their maximum extent.

References

British Paediatric Association (1994) *Services for Children and Adolescents with Learning Disability (Mental Handicap). Report of a British Paediatric Association Working Party.* British Paediatric Association, London.

Coppola G, Iervolino G, Mastrosimone M, La Torre G, Ruiu F and Poscotto A (2004) Melatonin in wake–sleep disorders in children, adolescents and young adults with mental retardation with or without epilepsy: a double-blind cross-over placebo-controlled trial. *Brain Dev.* **26:** 373–6.

Corbett J (1979) Psychiatric morbidity and mental retardation. In: FE James and RP Snaith (eds) *Psychiatric Illness and Mental Handicap.* Gaskell, London.

Gillberg C, Person E, Grumman M *et al.* (1986) Psychiatric disorders in mildly and severely mentally retarded urban children and adolescents: epidemiological aspects. *Br J Psychiatry.* **149:** 68–74.

Kiernan C and Quereshi H (1993) Challenging behaviour. In: C Kiernan (ed.) *Research to Practice? Implications of research on the challenging behaviour of people with learning disabilities.* British Institute of Learning Disabilities, Kidderminster.

Rutter M, Tizard J, Yule W *et al.* (1976) Isle of Wight Studies, 1964–74 Research Report. *Psychological Medicine.* **6:** 313–32.

Chapter 9

Psychiatric health and older people with intellectual disabilities

Mark Luty and Sally-Ann Cooper

Introduction

An ageing population

People with intellectual disability are an ageing population. In the past, few people with intellectual disability lived beyond childhood, whereas the majority can now expect to reach middle or old age. There are many reasons to account for this increase in lifespan. In part it reflects the increase in lifespan that has been seen for the whole population over the past century. However, there are factors that have had a greater impact for people with intellectual disability. These include improved access to medical treatments (e.g. surgery for congenital heart disease, antibiotics for chest infections), the move away from institutionalised living settings which potentiated the spread of infections such as tuberculosis, better lifestyles within the community, and more person-centred care enabling better nutrition, healthcare and social fulfilment. In the UK there are now more people with intellectual disability aged 40 years or over than there are children with learning disabilities. Older people with intellectual disability are increasing in number, and this trend will continue.

The increase in lifespan is occurring for people with intellectual disability of all types of causes and at all levels of ability. Despite this, the life expectancy of people with intellectual disability is still shorter than it is for the general population. Within the population of people with intellectual disability, some groups of people have a shorter life expectancy than others (e.g. those with Down syndrome, profound intellectual disability and multiple physical disabilities). The different life expectancies of specific groups mean that the population of older people with intellectual disability has different characteristics to the population of younger adults with intellectual disability. For example, people with more severe intellectual disability have a shorter life expectancy, so the population of older people has a comparatively less severe degree of intellectual disability overall.

Physical health

The pattern of physical health needs among older people with intellectual disability differs from that of younger adults with intellectual disability (NHS Scotland 2004). There are two main reasons for this. As the person with

107

intellectual disability ages, they have an increased risk of acquiring age-related physical health needs (e.g. due to arthritis, stroke and degenerative disorders). Some types of physical health needs are associated with the person's underlying cause of intellectual disability (e.g. as part of genetic syndromes, or neurological impairments). As there is a difference in the life expectancy of cohorts of adults with intellectual disability of specific causes, then for the whole population of adults with intellectual disability the profile of physical health needs differs with increasing age cohorts. In addition, the profile of physical health needs differs from that of the general population, as do the leading causes of death. Within the general population, the leading causes of death are cancer, followed by ischaemic heart disease, followed by stroke. For people with intellectual disability the leading causes of death are respiratory problems, followed by heart disease (congenital disease having greater prominence than ischaemic disease), and cancer is ranked lower (NHS Scotland 2004).

These differences in physical health needs are important in terms of both a person's individual management and public health strategies. An awareness of physical health need is also important when considering psychiatric ill health, as presenting symptoms can be the same for both psychiatric and physical ill health, especially in people with limited verbal communication skills. A change in behaviour, or the onset of problem behaviour, is an example of this. The rest of this chapter will focus on psychiatric ill health.

Social changes

There are social differences between the populations of older and younger adults with intellectual disability. Older adults will have had different life experiences and memories, different treatment histories and possibly different expectations compared with younger adults. Many will have spent some of their life (in some cases many decades from early infancy) living in institutions, as in the past this was the accepted model of care. In the past, educational opportunities were often limited. There may also have been less awareness in the past of exploitation and abuse and the consequences of stigma. These factors affect the way in which our personalities develop and the coping strategies that we adopt. As such they have an influence on a person's vulnerability to, or protection from, psychiatric health needs in adult life.

Prevalence of psychiatric ill health

One would expect older people with intellectual disability to have a high prevalence of psychiatric ill health. This is because, as well as experiencing the risk factors that affect the whole population (e.g. family genetic predisposition to major psychiatric disorders, life events, physical illnesses associated with psychiatric needs), they also have vulnerabilities due to factors associated with intellectual disability, and vulnerabilities related to older age. Examples are listed in Box 9.1.

> **Box 9.1: Additional vulnerability factors for psychiatric ill health**
>
> *Examples of vulnerability factors related to intellectual disabilities*
>
> - Behavioural phenotypes (e.g. Down syndrome, dementia and depression)
> - Epilepsy and neurological impairments
> - Multiple physical ill health and prescribed drugs
> - Adverse experiences in childhood (e.g. institutional care)
> - Adverse social circumstances (e.g. lack of choice, restricted social networks, lack of confidence, exploitation, abuse, stigma, poverty)
> - Developmental factors (e.g. communication difficulties) and patterns of behaviour related to a person's developmental age (e.g. head banging and tantrums)
>
> *Examples of vulnerability factors related to old age*
>
> - Neurological changes
> - Deterioration in physical health, resultant frailty and deteriorating mobility
> - Loss of confidence
> - Pain
> - Onset of sensory impairments
> - Bereavement and loss
> - Narrowing of social networks and activities

Older people with intellectual disability can develop the full range of psychiatric disorders. These can have onset during old age, or they may be longstanding disorders (e.g. pervasive developmental disorders, problem behaviours). Special factors to consider in the assessment of such disorders in older people include whether presentation of psychiatric illness is modified by physical frailty. Within the general population there have been several research projects exploring the different psychiatric presentations in older compared with younger adults. However, similar research has not yet been undertaken among people with intellectual disability.

There have been several studies of psychiatric ill health among older people with intellectual disability. There are difficulties in drawing comparisons between some studies due to biases in sample selection (e.g. some studies were based in hospitals or clinic populations), methods of assessment (e.g. some studies report known ill health whereas others comprehensively assessed study participants) and classification criteria.

There is a well-recognised association between Down syndrome and dementia, with almost all people with Down syndrome over the age of 40 years showing neuropathological changes (ß-amyloid plaques and neurofibrillary tangles) similar to those seen in dementia of Alzheimer's type (Mann 1988). However, clinical dementia is *not* an invariable consequence of Down syndrome, with only about 50% of all people with Down syndrome developing dementia by the time they have reached old age (Prasher 1995; Holland *et al.* 1998).

Dementia is prevalent among older people with intellectual disability, not just among people with Down syndrome. The studies of Lund (1985), Moss and Patel

Table 9.1 Prevalence of psychiatric ill health among older adults with intellectual disability

	Prevalence (%)
Dementia	22
Depression	6
Mania	0.7
Generalised anxiety disorder	9
Schizophrenia	3
Problem behaviours	15

(1993) and Cooper (1997a) are all population-based, and yield similar prevalence rates when age-matched (i.e. with dementia occurring in about 22% of people aged 65 years or over, and about 12% of people aged 50 years or over). These figures are much higher than those found in the age-matched general population. Corbett (1979) also noted a high rate of dementia in his population-based study, but did not cite prevalence. Conversely, Zigman *et al.* (2004) claim that standardised morbidity rates for dementia prevalence were not demonstrated to be different from those of the general population. However, their confidence intervals were wide. Their sample ascertainment and methods of assessment and classification of dementia differed from those employed in the above studies. Lack of previous attention to dementia among people with intellectual disability probably relates to the small number of older people with intellectual disability relative to the whole population of people with intellectual disability, and the focus of considerable clinical and research interest on the dementia of Down syndrome, which is typically experienced by adults under 65 years of age, due to differences in life expectancy.

Table 9.1 outlines the prevalence of some of the common types of psychiatric ill health found among older adults with intellectual disability (Cooper 1997b). Generalised anxiety disorders and depression are common. The prevalence of schizophrenia, obsessive-compulsive disorder, mania and autism is similar to that found in younger adults with intellectual disability. Lund (1985) found lower rates of anxiety and problem behaviour than were reported in the other studies. This may relate to the range of psychopathological items included in his data collection. The studies of Corbett (1979) and Cooper (1997a) allow comparisons of prevalence rates across age cohorts, and suggest that psychiatric health needs are greater in older than in younger adults with intellectual disability, particularly when dementia is included.

Psychiatric assessment

As a general rule, a change in the behaviour (adaptive behaviour or maladaptive behaviour) or well-being of a person with intellectual disability always indicates a health need (psychiatric or physical) until proven otherwise. Such changes may include the onset of a new symptom or a new behaviour, the exacerbation of a long-standing symptom or behaviour, or the cessation of a long-standing symptom or behaviour. Problem behaviour *never* has an onset in older age without there being an underlying health need (e.g. psychiatric illness such as dementia or depression, or physical ill health). Consequently, when there is a change in an older person's behaviour, this always requires referral for health assessment and treatment. The onset of some symptoms may easily be recognised by carers as requiring referral (e.g. a person complaining of hearing noises or voices when there is no one in the room to account for them (auditory hallucinations), or a normally calm person developing episodes of apparently unprovoked aggression). However, reductions in maladaptive behaviours can be just as significant with regard to understanding and assessing underlying psychiatric disorders (e.g. a person with Prader–Willi syndrome who starts to refuse food, or a usually boisterous person prone to shouting who becomes socially withdrawn and quiet).

Assessment of change is a key factor in psychiatric (and physical) health assessments. Consequently, eliciting background information from the past is essential in all psychiatric assessments. Although psychotic symptoms (delusions and hallucinations) are almost always abnormal and indicate the presence of psychiatric illness, they can occur in a number of different disorders and therefore require full assessment. Other types of symptoms may or may not be abnormal, depending on the person's usual state. For example, if a usually boisterous person starts to become socially withdrawn and quiet, this indicates a health need, whereas for another person being socially withdrawn and quiet may be an expression of their natural personality and indicate good health. Among the general population, in the majority of cases most symptoms may be considered to be indicative of ill health, whereas among the population of people with learning disabilities it is always essential to distinguish between state (i.e. new-onset) and trait (long-standing) symptoms/behaviour. The most often quoted example of this is the assessment of dementia. Assessing someone's level of adaptive skills cannot on its own be used to assess for the skills loss experienced in dementia, as people with intellectual disabilities have a wide range of baseline skill levels (depending on the degree of their intellectual disability and the extent of their education, training and practice of skills). Their current skill level has to be referred back to a previous reference level (i.e. the level at which they were functioning prior to any change in skills being noted). Some researchers advocate that assessment of change should be undertaken prospectively, but in clinical practice this is routinely undertaken retrospectively, using clinical judgement, as for all other types of symptom assessment for psychiatric ill health. Difficulties can arise when current carers have not known the person prior to the onset of problems (e.g. if the person has recently moved residential placements). In these situations, it is essential to trace further informants (e.g. from previous residential or day-care placements).

Psychiatric assessment looks for patterns of symptoms/behaviours (referenced back to the person's usual premorbid state), which is referred to as psychopathology. Symptoms that commonly occur in several psychiatric disorders include loss of skills, increase in or onset of aggression, poor concentration and social withdrawal. The full range of psychopathology that is found in the general population can be experienced by older people with intellectual disability, and determining its cause and from that the appropriate intervention/supports will be dependent on a comprehensive assessment. As carers/support workers may be more challenged in supporting a person who has onset of, for example, aggression or sleep disturbance, they are likely to report these symptoms spontaneously. It is essential that the assessing clinician routinely enquires about the full range of possible psychopathology, which will include possible symptoms that carers/support workers may not spontaneously describe or consider to be of importance. Carers/support workers may also fail to report symptoms due to diagnostic overshadowing (i.e. in settings for older people, carers may inadvertently interpret symptoms as part of a person's intellectual disabilities, and in intellectual disabilities settings, symptoms may be inadvertently interpreted as a normal feature of old age).

Box 9.2 summarises some of the key points in assessment of psychopathology/identification of a health need.

Box 9.2: Assessment of psychopathology/identification of a health need

- Change in behaviour indicates a health need and requires referral for health assessment.
- Both an increase and a decrease in existing behaviours can indicate a health need.
- Problem behaviour starting in old age always indicates underlying ill health.
- Assessment must always distinguish between long-standing (trait) and new-onset (state) behaviours/symptoms.
- When informants have not known the person with intellectual disability for long, information from further background informants will be required.
- The full range of psychiatric symptoms may occur in older adults with intellectual disability.
- Assessment of psychopathology must cover the full range of all possible psychopathology, not just that spontaneously reported by carers/support workers.
- People may misinterpret psychiatric symptoms as being due to intellectual disability or older age (diagnostic overshadowing).

Once the full range of psychopathology has been measured, it is classified using diagnostic criteria (a descriptive diagnosis). The descriptive diagnosis can have many underlying causes, and an integral part of psychiatric assessment includes differentiating the causes by assessing biological, psychological, social and developmental factors. As well as asking the person with intellectual disability and their carer about the current problems and clarifying the psychopathology, the assessment also covers past psychiatric illnesses and treatment, physical health (including problems in the past and a current review of all medical systems), drug assessment, health of family members, personal history (an account of important aspects of the person's life from birth through to the current time), their current social circumstances, developmental assessment (including the cause of the person's intellectual disability) and details of any forensic problems. Examinations include mental state and physical state, blood tests and sometimes other special investigations. This approach is necessarily different from and complementary to that of functional analysis, which will be familiar to some carers. Psychiatric diagnosis cannot be made on the basis of what happened today, or what happened in the last week, without reference to additional information from the past.

Comprehensive psychiatric assessments often include professionals from different disciplines working together (e.g. intellectual disability psychiatrists, intellectual disabilities nurses, psychologists, occupational therapists and social workers). It is essential for these professionals to develop good relationships with the person's carer/relative as well as the person with intellectual disability him- or herself, as assessment is very reliant on information from the carer/relative, as indeed is the implementation of management/treatment care plans and evaluation of their effectiveness, followed by appropriate revisions.

The differences between the techniques employed in psychiatric assessment and management when working with someone of average ability and when working with someone with intellectual disability are described in more detail elsewhere (Cooper 2003).

Dementia

Types of dementia

Dementia is common in middle-aged people with Down syndrome, and in older people with intellectual disability of other causes. It is an age-related disorder (i.e. it increases in prevalence with increasing age), and can have several underlying causes. The commonest types are dementia in Alzheimer's disease, dementia with Lewy bodies and vascular dementia. Skill loss and cognitive loss are features common to all types of dementia. Some less common causes of dementia are potentially reversible (e.g. vitamin B_{12} deficiency), so differential diagnosis is important. Determining the cause of the dementia presentation leads to identification of the most appropriate plan for interventions/supports.

Presentation of dementia

There are a number of symptoms and signs that can occur as a feature of dementia. A person with dementia will have some but not all of these symptoms, so each person's presentation may be slightly different. As the dementia progresses, skill loss and symptoms increase. Symptoms include the following.

- The person may require more prompting than was previously necessary to complete tasks, or may only half-complete tasks that used to be completed.
- The person may have difficulty following instructions as well as they did in the past, and may require these to be broken down into smaller component parts.
- All types of skills can be affected (e.g. literacy, financial skills, dressing, washing, cleaning, cooking, communication, understanding, continence, feeding skills and social skills). Skill loss is progressive.
- The individual may develop problems with their recent memory (e.g. forgetting what they have done at work that day or what they have just eaten, bringing the wrong bag or coat home, or mislaying possessions).
- Memory from the more distant past remains more intact in the early stages of dementia. Sometimes the person will talk about the past as if it is the present (e.g. they may mention living with their parents although the latter may have died some years ago).

- Increased disorientation with regard to place and time may also occur. For example, a person who used to find their way around at their day centre may become unable to do so, getting lost or wandering off aimlessly into the street, or a person who used to be able to keep track of time may lose track of it (e.g. getting up in the middle of the night and insisting that it is time to get dressed and go out).
- The person may become dyspraxic (e.g. putting their clothes on back to front when this was a task that they used to be able to complete competently).
- Judgement and decision making become increasingly impaired.
- The person loses the ability to walk, and weight loss may occur.
- The person may develop neurological signs such as seizures, primitive reflexes, and when lying in bed adopting a position in which the head is slightly raised (psychogenic pillow).
- Non-cognitive symptoms of dementia are also common. They include psychotic symptoms, such as visual hallucinations of strangers in the house and persecutory delusions. Auditory hallucinations can also occur. Other common non-cognitive symptoms of dementia include apathy, loss of energy, anxiety and agitation, aggression, loss of concentration, sleep disturbance and reduced social interaction.

The rate of progress of these symptoms is variable, and the first symptoms that are seen will depend on the person's original level of intellectual disabilities (e.g. if they have never been able to identify coins, then onset of dementia will not be associated with loss of financial skills).

Assessment of dementia

If a person with intellectual disability starts to lose skills, or develops any other changes as outlined above, it is important that they are referred for a comprehensive health assessment. The purpose of this is to establish the descriptive diagnosis, determine its causes and set up appropriate intervention/support care plans to maximise the person's functioning. Some of the differential diagnoses to be considered when assessing dementia are outlined in Box 9.3.

Box 9.3: Some differential diagnoses to consider when assessing dementia

- Toxic (e.g. drugs, infection, poisons)
- Metabolic (e.g. thyroid disease)
- Respiratory disease – either from the effects of disease (e.g. neoplasia) or the result of disease (e.g. hypoxia)
- Cardiovascular (e.g. cerebrovascular accident, hypertension)
- Haematological (e.g. anaemia)
- Neurological (e.g. hydrocephalus, epilepsy)
- Nutritional (e.g. vitamin B_{12} or folate deficiency, obesity)
- Sleep disturbance – sleep apnoea
- Sensory – hearing loss and visual impairment
- Gastrointestinal (e.g. neoplasia)
- Psychiatric (e.g. depression, bereavement, psychosis)
- Social (e.g. changes in environment or expectations)

Assessment includes taking a full history (as described above). The psychopathology assessment includes all symptoms of dementia, as well as symptoms of other psychiatric disorders which can mimic dementia (e.g. depression and schizophrenia). The review of medical systems includes questions about physical disorders that can mimic dementia, while the social assessment component of the psychiatric history may be of particular importance with regard to planning the person's further care. After the full psychiatric/medical history has been taken, a mental state examination, full physical examination and investigations are completed. A computed tomography (CT) or magnetic resonance imaging (MRI) head scan may be undertaken to exclude focal neurological lesions or hydrocephalus (but it is not yet possible to diagnose dementia from these scans, particularly in people with intellectual disability in whom abnormal scan findings are often found, related to the person's underlying cause of intellectual disabilities). Other investigations may be indicated, depending on the findings of the above assessments, scans, etc.

Box 9.4: Assessment of dementia

- Full psychiatric history, including measurement of psychopathology, past medical history, drugs, family history, personal history, social history and developmental history
- Physical health history
- Mental state examination
- Physical examination, including hearing and vision
- Full blood count
- Erythrocyte sedimentation rate or C-reactive protein
- Urea and electrolytes
- Blood glucose level
- Liver function tests
- Serum vitamin B_{12} and red cell folate
- Thyroid function tests
- Syphilis serology (if indicated)
- Chest X-ray
- A midstream urine sample sent for microscopy and culture
- Electrocardiogram
- CT or MRI head scan (if indicated)
- Other special investigations (if indicated)

At the end of this process it should be possible to attribute a descriptive diagnosis to the person's symptoms and signs, and when this is dementia, to determine the probable causes and the contributions made by various factors. The next stage is to set up the intervention/support care plans.

Management of dementia

There are several important stages to the management of dementia. This is often undertaken by several professionals from different disciplines working together. It is essential that the carer/relative of the person concerned is fully consulted and involved and their agreement to the plans sought, as well as that of the person with intellectual disability (as far as he or she has capacity to understand).

Correction of any treatable disorders or problems

This depends on the findings of the assessment and might include, for example, correcting a thyroid disorder, treatment for anaemia, a hearing assessment and provision of a hearing aid, cutting very overgrown toenails to aid walking, and changing drug regimes in order to minimise drug side-effects. Correction of these problems helps to maximise functional ability.

Reducing vulnerability factors with regard to dementia

A person with early vascular dementia or a history suggesting a high risk of developing this disorder might benefit from reducing risk factors (e.g. by dietary changes with a view to weight loss and cholesterol reduction, giving up smoking, relaxation, antihypertensive drugs to reduce blood pressure, and regular treatment with aspirin). Consideration might also be given to the use of hormonal treatment, non-steroidal anti-inflammatory agents and antioxidants.

Treating non-cognitive symptoms of dementia

A range of treatment strategies might be employed for non-cognitive symptoms of dementia, depending on their underlying cause. For example, aggression might be secondary to persecutory delusions or hallucinations, in which case antipsychotic drugs may be indicated, although treatment must be cautious in individuals with risk factors for cerebrovascular disease. Alternatively, in individuals with severe anxiety disorders, relaxation and distraction techniques as well as anxiolytic drugs may be helpful. Depending on the person's level of intellectual disability, relaxation techniques may necessarily have to involve semi-hypnotic approaches, or the use of massage, aromatherapy, bubble baths/foot spas, Snoezelen rooms or soft music. If aggression is due to 'catastrophic' reactions in which seemingly small events stretch the person to beyond the limit of their understanding and coping mechanisms, the appropriate management is likely to be the provision of education and advice to the carer/relative in managing daily tasks and situations, together with the offer of adequate support/respite care. Effective treatments can be offered for many of the non-cognitive symptoms of dementia, provided that they have been adequately assessed. Some people in the early stages of dementia have an awareness of their skill loss, memory changes and changes to thought processes. This may be distressing or confusing, and the person may benefit from individual time to discuss and explore these experiences and any fears that they may have.

Behavioural management of cognitive symptoms of dementia

Behavioural management can be helpful and might include, for example, the use of pictorial daily planners to help the person to orientate him- or herself through the events of the day, labelling doors with pictures to aid orientation, the use of pictorial communication boards, and reminiscent groups (perhaps using life-story books). Routine and repetition can be helpful.

Drug treatment of cognitive symptoms of dementia

In the UK four drugs are licensed at present for the treatment of dementia in Alzheimer's disease (donepezil, rivastigmine, galantamine and memantine). These have been evaluated in people with intellectual disability and dementia, but only on a very limited scale (Prasher 2004). The extent to which they are or are not beneficial will become clearer in future.

Education

It is important to offer an explanation both to the person with intellectual disability and to their relative/carer. This will involve explaining the diagnosis, discussing the future and possible future care needs, and describing the available support services. The emotional impact of this information is likely to be such that several sessions may be required, and the pace at which information is imparted should be gauged individually and with sensitivity. If relatives/carers are well informed this may help their decision making with regard to future planning and may also help them emotionally.

Carer support

Caring for a person with intellectual disability who is losing skills can be stressful, particularly when he or she is a much-loved relative. Emotional support may be beneficial – for example, a professional with whom feelings such as loss can be discussed, and with whom concerns and fears can be shared. Practical support is important. For example, establishment of regular respite care may be helpful. Some carers/relatives find contact with their local voluntary organisation helpful (e.g. the Alzheimer's Society, Age Concern or Mencap). Some voluntary organisations provide useful leaflet information for carers, hold support groups where people in similar situations can share experiences, and provide care services.

Social aspects of care

As a person's needs change, their support packages and benefits will require review and modification. Opportunities for recreation and occupation are important, particularly if they allow the person the opportunities to practise skills in a supportive, non-threatening, non-pressured environment (the longer skills are used, possibly the longer they will be retained). Such opportunities are important to enable the person to continue to maintain a high quality of life. As the dementia progresses, the person's support needs will increase, and so to enable the person to continue to age – and ultimately die – at home, increased support provision will need to be provided within his or her home.

Management of psychiatric disorders other than dementia

The framework outlined above for the management of dementia can also be used, with modification, for other types of psychiatric ill health. There are some considerations that are more relevant to older people than to younger people with intellectual disability. As people age, their metabolism changes, which affects drug pharmacokinetics. This often means that older people appear to be more 'sensitive' to drug side-effects. Coexisting age-related disease can also increase the likelihood of adverse reactions to drugs. For example, a person with dementia (even in the very early stages before this has been diagnosed) is more likely to develop acute confusional states (delirium) in response to many classes of drugs (including several psychotropic drugs).

Other management strategies (e.g. behavioural interventions) also need to be sensitive to the person's age and physical health. Many older people would not consider a trip out to a disco or nightclub or a long shopping trip to be a reward (although some might). Many older people would not welcome a hectic, noisy work placement (although some would). Many older people might prefer to work and socialise with peers of a similar age to themselves (although some would prefer to mix with younger people).

With these considerations in mind, standard intellectual disability psychiatric intervention/support plans should be employed for older people to meet their psychiatric health needs as identified by the assessment.

Services and supports

Previous work has found that people with intellectual disability encounter barriers to accessing appropriate healthcare. This is true for older people as well as younger adults.

Service provision for people with intellectual disability has changed in recent years, following the move from institutional care to community care. For some older people this may mean that they have to adapt to a substantial change if until recently they have only known life within an institution. Models of service provision differ in different countries, but long-stay institutional closure is being implemented across the developed world. Older people with intellectual disability living in the community are likely to require provision of support and care from teams of support workers. They may also require support from professionals from a range of disciplines, sometimes working as part of a multi-disciplinary team. Local communities may also be an important source of support. It may be confusing for the older person to understand the different roles that are provided when multiple professionals are involved in their care and support. This is particularly important at times of change (e.g. the common scenario following the death of an elderly parent who was the person's main carer).

Older people with intellectual disability access services and supports from a range of providers. Some facilities are designed for use by adults with intellectual disability, while others are designed primarily for use by the older general population. In both of these settings older people with intellectual disability will be in a minority. There is potential for inexperienced care staff in intellectual disability settings to inadvertently interpret the health needs of the older person as 'normal' for old age, and therefore not to refer the person for healthcare. Similarly, inexperienced care staff in facilities designed for use by older people may inadvertently interpret the health needs of the person with intellectual disability as a 'normal' component of the intellectual disability, and so not refer the person for healthcare. Table 9.2 outlines some of the services and supports that an older person with intellectual disability may require.

The organisation of services will vary in different localities. Within a locality, it is important that there is a clearly identified lead agency/officer responsible for the needs of older people with intellectual disability. This lead might be provided from older people's services or intellectual disability services, and will necessarily require collaboration between the two. The lead should be responsible for undertaking local health needs assessment for this population, identification of service gaps, and service planning, as well as for organisation and delivery of

Table 9.2 Services and supports for older people with intellectual disability

Health services	Social services and community supports
General practitioner	Social worker
Practice nurse	Home carers
Intellectual disability psychiatrist	Advocate
Old age psychiatrists	Support workers
Physician (e.g. cardiologist, neurologist)	Relatives
Psychologist	Voluntary or charitable organisations
Community intellectual disability nurse	Community workers
Community psychiatric nurse	Neighbours
District nurse	Community police
Continence nurse	Day-centre workers
Occupational therapist	Housing Association
Physiotherapist	
Speech and language therapist	
Dietitian	
Podiatrist	
Swallowing therapist	
Optician	
Dentist	

services and supports. This may help to reduce barriers to accessing services, and lead to better-coordinated service provision and delivery.

References

Cooper S-A (1997a) High prevalence of dementia amongst elderly people with learning disabilities not attributable to Down's syndrome. *Psychol Med.* **27:** 609–16.

Cooper S-A (1997b) Epidemiology of psychiatric disorders in elderly compared with younger adults with learning disabilities. *Br J Psychiatry.* **170:** 375–80.

Cooper S-A (2003) Classification and assessment in learning disability. *Psychiatry.* **2:** 12–17.

Corbett JA (1979) Psychiatric morbidity and mental retardation. In: FE James and RP Snaith (eds) *Psychiatric Illness and Mental Handicap.* Gaskell Press, London.

Holland AJ, Hon J, Huppert FA, Stevens F and Watson P (1998) Population-based study of the prevalence and presentation of dementia in adults with Down's syndrome. *Br J Psychiatry.* **172:** 493–8.

Lund J (1985) The prevalence of psychiatric morbidity in mentally retarded adults. *Acta Psychiatr Scand.* **72:** 565–70.

Mann DMA (1988) Alzheimer's disease and Down's syndrome. *Histopathology.* **13:** 125–37.

Moss S and Patel P (1993) The prevalence of mental illness in people with intellectual disability over 50 years of age, and the diagnostic importance of information from carers. *Ir J Psychol.* **14:** 110–29.

NHS Scotland (2004) *People with Learning Disabilities in Scotland. Health Needs Assessment Report.* NHS Scotland, Glasgow.

Prasher VP (1995) Age-specific prevalence, thyroid dysfunction and depressive symptomatology in adults with Down's syndrome and dementia. *Int J Geriatr Psychiatry.* **10:** 25–31.

Prasher VP (2004) Review of donepezil, rivastigmine, galantamine and memantine for the treatment of dementia in Alzheimer's disease in adults with Down syndrome: implications for the intellectual disability population. *Int J Geriatr Psychiatry.* **19:** 509–15.

Zigman WB, Schupf N, Devanny DA *et al.* (2004) Incidence and prevalence of dementia in elderly adults with mental retardation without Down syndrome. *Am J Ment Retard.* **109:** 126–41.

Chapter 10

Sexuality and people with intellectual disabilities

Meera Roy

Introduction

Sexuality relates to how people express themselves as men and women. This is culturally defined and influenced by family, peers, religion, the law, customs, knowledge and economics. Development of sexual maturity is a biological process which happens to almost everyone, including people with a learning disability (the exceptions include people with syndromes that affect sexual maturation). Heshusius (1987) reviewed the literature on perceptions of sexuality by people with learning disabilities and found that 'at least for the most part, sex is desirable, an essential part of life, pleasurable and adding warmth and excitement to living – not unlike the meaning it carries for most people'. In this chapter we shall examine how society has responded to people with learning disabilities expressing their sexuality, and the particular issues which face them in the areas of sex education, abuse, contraception and parenthood.

Historical overview

The concept of the expression of sexuality by people with a learning disability has caused unease in society in general and carers in particular from very early times. Until recent years, the response has been to lock them away in institutions where the care practices allowed little scope for appropriate sexual behaviour. *Eugenics* is the term applied to theories and practices ostensibly designed to improve the human condition in terms of genetics. However, the identification of desirable human traits is a subjective matter. References to eugenic ideals appear in the Old Testament, and Plato's *Republic* idealises a society in which there is a constant selection for the improvement of human stock.

In the UK, the Eugenic Education Society was set up in the early part of the twentieth century, drawing its membership from the middle classes, and it was most concerned by the growing problem presented by the 'feeble minded'. In response to increasing pressure, a Royal Commission was set up under the Chairmanship of the Earl of Radnor in 1904, which deliberated for 4 years. The Commission came to the conclusion that heredity was an important factor in 'mental deficiency', that 'defectives' were often highly prolific, and that other social problems such as delinquency and alcoholism were aggravated by the fact that so many 'defectives' were allowed complete freedom of action in the community. However, the Commission was not willing to consider sterilisation as an option, and insisted that the main criterion for certification should be the protection and happiness of the 'defective' rather than the purification of the race. In 1910, members of the Eugenic Society and the National Association for the Care of the Feeble-Minded lobbied the candidates for the General Election, asking them to support prevention of parenthood for the feeble-minded. However, the Mental Deficiency Act of 1913 did not address the issue of sterilisation.

A joint committee of the Board of Education and the Board of Control under the chairmanship of A H Wood in 1924 was asked to determine how many 'feeble-minded' people there were and how to deal with them. They concluded that the real criterion of 'mental deficiency' was social inefficiency and not educational subnormality, and they laid down principles of care. They recommended segregation and sterilisation for the elimination of individuals with 'primary amentia'. A Department of Health Committee chaired by L G Brock in 1934 recommended sterilisation for 'mentally defectives' with third-party consent, but this recommendation was not acted upon.

In the USA, the American Eugenics Society was founded in 1926 by men who believed that the white race was superior to other races, and that the upper classes had superior hereditary qualities that justified their being the ruling class. The sterilisation and segregation of 'defective' individuals was thought to be the best way to improve society. By 1931, sterilisation laws had been enacted by 27 states in the USA, and by 1935 similar laws had been passed in Denmark, Switzerland, Germany, Norway and Sweden. In most cases the purpose was clearly eugenic, although some laws tacitly permitted sterilisation for social rather than genetic reasons.

Following the atrocities in Hitler's Germany during the Second World War, the Eugenic Movement fell into disgrace. In 1942 in *Skinner v Oklahoma* the US Supreme Court ruling was that 'the right to procreate is a basic constitutional one', demonstrating a diametrically opposite view to that expressed by Oliver Wendell Holmes 1927 in the same court, in *Buck v Bell*, namely that 'three generations of imbeciles are enough'.

Sterilisation and people with learning disabilities

Once the eugenic argument is put aside, there still remain family or carer issues that impinge on the sexual rights of this group of people. Adults with learning disability may be looked upon as children and therefore viewed as asexual. Alternatively, they may be regarded as people with an excessive sexual drive and poor personal control. Parents give a variety of reasons for seeking to have their children with learning disabilities sterilised. Some feel that irresponsible behaviour on the part of their daughters will lead to their sexual exploitation. Others dread the possible emotional and economic burden of bringing up a child resulting from such a sexual encounter. There is a common belief that their daughter's disability would be transmitted to the next generation. Some parents favour sterilisation because they believe that it would result in a lowering of sexual drive. Others do so because they fear the social stigma that would result from their daughter becoming pregnant and the possibility of this being attributed to insufficient control and supervision on their part. Most requests for sterilisation come not from women with learning disabilities but from their parents, who feel that they have a right to be free from worry about their offspring beyond a certain age. Parents sometimes also cite their grandchildren's right to be born without disabilities.

In recent years, such cases have come into the public domain, leading to the clarification of the legal situation in England and Wales. In the case of minors, such an operation should only be performed with the permission of the High Court Judge obtained in wardship proceedings. In the case of adults over the age of 18 years who cannot give consent, the operation should be in their best interests and should be in accordance with the responsible body of medical opinion. The doctor performing the operation must consult all of the relevant professionals and family members, and should apply to the Court for a Declaration that, under the facts of the case, the operation would be lawful (Whitfield 1989).

In Scotland the law is different, as childhood is divided into two phases following the Roman Law classification of persons. There are *pupils*, who are protected and controlled by *tutors* (normally the parents) who have full control (subject to the welfare principle) over the pupil's property and person, and there are *minors* (between the ages of 12 or 14 and 18 years), who are protected by *curators* who only have control over the child's property. A tutor has the right to decide on medical treatment for the child, and a tutor dative can be appointed by the Sessions Court to consent to medical treatment for an adult so long as it is in his or her best interests (McK Norrie 1989).

In the USA, at present there appear to be three different approaches to sterilisation in the different states. In some states the operation cannot be performed on a person who cannot give consent. In the second group, the Court can evaluate cases for sterilisation and authorise the procedure if it is considered to be in the person's best interests. The third approach is to leave the decision to members of the family and their physician without resort to the courts (Annas 1981). In Canada, the Supreme Court concluded that 'non-therapeutic' sterilisations cannot be authorised by a Court (McKnorrie 1989). In Australia, in the state of Victoria all sterilisation operations have to be referred to the Guardianship tribunal (Carney and Singer 1986).

Sex education

The sterilisation of people with a learning disability may be seen as an extreme reaction to their sexuality. In the last few years their sexuality has been viewed more positively and there has been increasing public awareness of the right of people with learning disabilities to be treated like others without such disabilities, as a result of the pioneering work by Wolfensberger in the context of normal-isation or social role valorisation. In 1979, the United Nations adopted a Declaration of the Rights of the Mentally Handicapped, which states that 'the mentally retarded have the same basic rights as other citizens of the same country and same age'.

Craft (1987) believed that people with learning disabilities have six main rights with regard to their sexuality:

- the right to grow up and to be treated with the respect and dignity accorded to adults. This is often compromised due to their need for some level of support. All too often the support given has the effect of encouraging dependence

- the right to know – that is, to have access to as much information about themselves and their bodies and those of other people, their emotions, appropriate social behaviour, etc., as they can assimilate
- the right to be sexual and to make and break relationships
- the right not to be at the mercy of the individual sexual attitudes of different caregivers
- the right not to be sexually abused
- the right to a humane and dignified environment.

The Human Rights Act (1998) also has implications for people with a learning disability. Article 12 concerns the right to marry – that is, that men and women of marriageable age have the right to marry and found a family – which should be considered in relation to people with a learning disability. They also have a right to private and family life under Article 8. However, they would need appropriate education in the arena of sexuality and personal relationships to be able to meet these objectives.

In the last decade, there have been improvements in the provision of sex education both for the general population and for people with learning disabilities. The attitudes of staff in residential settings have become more progressive in moving towards an acceptance of a socio-sexual life for the people in their care (Heshusius 1987). Those who receive sex education appear to benefit substantially in terms of knowledge, growth and self-confidence (Robinson 1987). Without this, they will be unable to develop meaningful relationships.

As the majority of people with learning disabilities live with parents or paid carers, such carers have an important role to play in allowing the development and expression of sexuality. When planning sex education, it is important that parents and carers are consulted at an early stage. Training staff to deal appropriately with sexuality is essential in order to prevent traditional repressive reactions. Training must be on at least two levels. First, all staff need awareness training in order to develop awareness that individuals with a learning disability have needs and rights with regard to their sexuality. They also need information on a range of issues such as local services, availability of educational materials, pregnancy, etc. Secondly, a small number of staff may want to undertake further training to work as teachers and counsellors themselves. Various organisations (e.g. the British Institute of Learning Disabilities, the Association to Aid the Personal and Sexual Relationships of People with Learning Disabilities, and the Education and Training Department of the Family Planning Association) run such courses (Craft and Brown 1994). There are training packs (e.g. *Not a Child Anymore*, produced by the Brook Advisory Service) which can be used to provide sex education for people with learning disabilities.

Issues of personal relationships and sexuality are now being addressed in schools for children with a learning disability.

An important prerequisite for effective sex education is an awareness and understanding of one's own attitudes, beliefs and practices both with regard to sexuality and towards people with learning disabilities. Those providing the service must be sensitive to the needs of minority groups such as Asian and African-Caribbean people, and guard against negative stereotypes (e.g. that black people and those with learning disabilities have strong sexual desires) (Baxter 1994).

People with learning disabilities as parents

In 1942 the US Supreme Court stated that the right to procreate was a basic constitutional right. Sterilisation would forever deprive a person of this right, which is fundamental to the existence and survival of the human race. In 1987 the Law Lords considered that the presence of physical and mental disability in a girl rendered her incapable of ever exercising that right or enjoying that privilege.

Tymchuk and Andron (1994) reviewed a large body of literature on people with learning disabilities functioning as parents. The main drawbacks of the studies were as follows.

1 They concerned deinstitutionalised people, so caution must be exercised with regard to generalising the findings to people raised and living in the community.
2 The parents studied were not representative of the general population, as they had been referred by the courts.
3 There was a general lack of sophistication, with a lack of comparability of methodology.

There appeared to be no clear evidence to suggest that people with learning disabilities predominantly gave birth to children with learning disabilities. However, as many of these people lived in impoverished environments, it is difficult to determine the effects of poverty as opposed to being brought up by parents with disabilities. Yet Gillberg and Geijer-Karlsson (1983) found that women with learning disabilities had more children compared with the general population, and that they also had more children with learning disabilities. Women with learning disabilities who do well as mothers have the following traits: adequate reading and comprehension abilities to enable them to use traditional sources of information such as parenting manuals; IQ above 60; no concomitant emotional disturbance; no concomitant medical disorders; low stress levels; adequate self-concept; adequate motivation. Good outcome is also associated with the following environmental factors: only one child in the house; having a younger child; having a child without medical or other problems; having a partner without an emotional disorder, criminal behaviour or behaviour problems, including abuse of spouse; having sufficient supports (social, health, financial, vocational, psychological and legal); not having been institutionalised; having had their own appropriate role models during their own upbringing; having adequately trained professionals; availability and appropriateness of materials used in training; continuity of agency; having a single agency providing multiple services and/or coordination (Tymchuk *et al.* 1990).

Normal intelligence does not guarantee good parenting skills. Conversely, the presence of learning disabilities does not preclude the ability to be a good parent. If a person with learning disabilities is to be a parent, they should be assessed to find out their strengths and areas where they are likely to need help. Under the current legislation, the child's needs must be paramount. Early assessment and planned intervention are essential to ensure that there is as little disruption as possible for the child and the parents with learning disability. Parenting skills can be assessed in family centres where people with learning disabilities can also receive training in childcare. Psychologists and psychiatrists working in the field of learning disability may be called upon to give expert opinion on cognitive abilities and the presence of psychiatric disorders which may affect the ability to parent. There should be close liaison between community learning disability teams supporting the person with learning disabilities, childcare teams, family centre staff, partners, the person with learning disabilities and any involved family member. If the decision is made that the individual can cope with parenthood, the next step is to put together a comprehensive package to cover the period leading up to delivery and the postnatal period. The parent with learning disabilities may need help and support over a long period of time to help them to deal with the child's developmental stages. However, if it appears that they are likely to put the child at risk either during the initial assessment or at any time subsequently, it will be necessary to implement childcare proceedings.

In their book *Parenting Under Pressure*, Tim and Wendy Booth (Booth and Booth 1994) describe their work with parents with learning disabilities. They suggest that much has still to be learned in this field, particularly on achieving a balance between the welfare of the children and the rights of the parents. All too often the balance is tipped against the parents. Although children must be protected, it is important that parents with learning disabilities are not abused by the system. Prosser (1992) defined a number of characteristics of 'system abuse' of parents, based on their perceptions of the treatment that they had received at the hands of child protection agencies. These include actions that harm the people whom they are supposed to help, snap judgements made on the basis of inadequate evidence, failing to involve people in decisions that affect them, adding to the problems already facing them, seeing people in isolation from their close relationships, and treating people as ciphers. Booth and Booth (1994) suggest a set of guidelines for practitioners working with parents with learning disabilities which are useful to adopt in order to reduce prejudicial attitudes and misconceptions. It is important that workers in child protection agencies have a good understanding of people with learning disabilities if the latter are to have a chance of succeeding as parents. However, even practitioners who are sympathetic find themselves trapped by the system into taking actions or decisions that oppress learning-disabled individuals. This suggests that there may be a need to change the service system itself.

The government White Paper *Valuing People: a new strategy for learning disability for the twenty-first century* (Department of Health 2001) has acknowledged that support for disabled parents is patchy and underdeveloped, with tensions and conflicts within social services departments between those whose focus is the welfare of the child and those who are concerned with the parent. It identified the Director of Social Services as being responsible for ensuring effective partnership working for parents with learning disabilities between children's and adult teams. Partnership Boards are responsible for ensuring that services are available to support parents with a learning disability. The work in this area must be ongoing if parents with a learning disability are to be successful. Most parents with learning disabilities are likely to find parenting an uphill task. However, they can succeed if they are given the right kind of support.

Around the UK there are organisations which provide specialist support services for parents with a learning disability in addition to the family centres run by social services. When presented with a parent with a learning disability it may be useful to obtain specialist input from one of them.

Contraceptive options

On the whole, people with learning disabilities have the same range of contraceptive options as the general population, and the choice of contraceptive depends on the person's individual circumstances. From a review of the menstrual and contraceptive options offered to young women attending her gynaecology clinic between 1990 and 1999, Grover (2002) has shown that the management is similar to that in women without a disability.

Natural family planning methods (e.g. only having intercourse during the safe period) require motivation, knowledge and planning on the part of the users. This is not a foolproof method for most people, including those with learning disabilities. Barrier methods (e.g. condoms) may be suitable for people with mild learning disabilities who are motivated to have good contraception without the need to take tablets. Absence of coexisting personality disorders with poor impulse control and physical disabilities that compromise manual dexterity would increase the success rate of these methods.

Intrauterine devices (IUDs) are highly effective, have no metabolic side-effects, and only a single act of motivation is required for long-term use. Once *in situ* they only need to be checked annually. They are often used by women who have borne children, as side-effects such as painful periods and heavy blood loss occur less often than in nulliparous women. Devices containing progesterone are said to cause less menstrual blood loss. Intrauterine devices are suitable for women with mild learning disabilities who may have problems remembering to take the pill every day. This is often the reason why women without a disability choose to use IUDs. They may also be suitable for women with severe learning disabilities who are unable to take oral contraceptive pills because of the side-effects. However, heavier menstruation may exacerbate any hygiene-related problems, and a general anaesthetic may be necessary, both for the insertion and for annual checks. In view of the risk of removal by the woman or her partner, shorter threads on the device and more frequent checks may be advisable. The use of IUDs is generally inadvisable in nulliparous women, due to the increased risk of pelvic infection and infertility.

The oral contraceptive pill would be the method of choice for women with mild learning disabilities who are motivated to have a safe, efficient system of contraception. It can also be used by women with more severe degrees of learning disability who are given their medication by their carers. A higher dose of the combined (oestrogen and progestogen) pill may be necessary if the woman is concurrently taking an anticonvulsant that induces liver enzymes. Injectable depot preparations of progesterone may be useful for women with mild learning disabilities for short periods of time if compliance is poor and an IUD is not appropriate. It may also be useful for women with severe learning disabilities, for whom a general anaesthetic may be unsuitable due to other physical problems. Amenorrhoea, which frequently occurs with long-term use, may be beneficial. Careful counselling is required to ensure that the woman is able to give informed consent.

Sterilisation (consisting of tubal ligation for women and vasectomy for men) is a safe and permanent method of contraception. Voluntary sterilisation of either partner is the most frequently used method of fertility regulation in the world. Men and women with mild learning disabilities who have completed their families and are able to give informed consent can make use of this option. Women with severe learning disabilities who are unable to consent but are sexually active and unable to use other options such as the pill or IUD because of side-effects can also have sterilisation, so long as the doctor performing the surgery has followed the guidelines outlined earlier in this chapter. The relatively permanent nature of sterilisation and the issue of informed consent are the main drawbacks.

Consent

Informed consent is an essential prerequisite for any treatment. The various components are as follows.

- It must be voluntary and obtained without misrepresentation or fraud.
- The act performed must be consistent with the act for which consent was obtained.
- The act must not in itself be illegal.
- The person must be given sufficient information regarding the purpose, nature and consequences of the proposed treatment to enable them to make a reasoned decision as to whether to accept or reject the treatment.
- The person must have the legal capacity (age and mental competence) to give consent.

Mental competence is defined as the ability of the intellect to meet a challenge. In people with learning disabilities it can be difficult to ascertain the degree of competence, to know if a reasoned decision has been reached and to establish whether it is truly voluntary. If the learning disability is severe, there is often a total incapacity to communicate and give consent. In the past, in these circumstances third-party consent has been obtained from parents or guardians, and from a court in the case of children. This is acceptable in situations in which the person's life is at risk, but becomes untenable when the issue is potentially irreversible control of fertility. The current legal status is that parents, guardians or the court can consent on behalf of a person with learning disabilities up to the age of 18 years for treatments excluding those that would interfere with fertility. Beyond this age, no one can give consent on behalf of another. The law regarding sterilisation has been discussed earlier in the chapter.

Sexual abuse of people with learning disabilities

Like other people with disabilities, those with learning disabilities have been shown to be at greater risk of sexual abuse. Browning and Boatman (1977) found that 14% of incest victims had intellectual disabilities. Elvik *et al.* (1990) physically examined 35 girls and women (aged 13–55 years) with mental retardation and found that 37% of these cases had clear physical evidence of sexual abuse, an additional 6% had a known history of sexual assaults and a further 6% had sexually transmitted diseases.

People with learning disabilities are at increased risk of abuse because of their dependence on other people for personal care, an imbalance of power between the person being cared for and the carer, difficulties in communication, lack of sexual knowledge and assertiveness, and guilt and shame about being disabled

(Sinason 1993a,b). Turk and Brown (1993) found that the victims were usually women and the perpetrators were usually men, and that the perpetrator was often known to the victim. Many perpetrators abuse more than one victim.

The victim of abuse may present with changes in personality or behaviour, sexually inappropriate behaviour, withdrawal, sleep disturbance, loss of skills or reduced level of functioning, loss of or reduction in speech, self-injurious behaviour or symptoms of post-traumatic stress disorder. To date there have been very few successful prosecutions against perpetrators. Many cases do not get to court because the Crown Prosecution Service or the police consider a person with learning disabilities to be an unreliable witness (Cooke and Sinason 1998).

Children and adults with mental and physical disabilities face particular difficulties when trying to tell of abuse. They are more likely to be disbelieved or even ignored. Their communication problems are exploited by their abuser, who is subtly aided by many of the unthinking networks in which they exist. The therapists are often disadvantaged, too, as they may not have skills in the field of learning disabilities. The communication problem of the person with learning disabilities may be further compounded by the emotional trauma of abuse. Body language may be used to communicate sexual abuse (e.g. excessive masturbation or eroticised inappropriate behaviour) (Sinason 1994).

Various psychotherapeutic approaches have been modified to treat the victims of abuse. Psychiatric illness (e.g. depression) precipitated by sexual abuse should be treated with appropriate medication. Defects in cognitive functioning may make it difficult to process memories and emotions induced by the abuse, leading to chronic psychological dysfunctioning (Cooke and Sinason 1998). Professionals working in the field of learning disability should be aware of the possibility of sexual abuse. It is recommended that health and social service units have procedures to deal with alleged sexual abuse.

The Royal College of Psychiatrists in collaboration with St George's Hospital has brought out *Books Beyond Words* to help people with learning disabilities to talk about their experiences. The series includes books dealing with sexual abuse (Hollins and Sinason 2005). Organisations such as Respond and the Ann Craft Trust provide training both in working with people who have been abused and in preventing abuse.

People with learning disabilities as sex offenders

It is commonly agreed that deviant sexual behaviour is similar for disabled and non-disabled offenders (Sinason 1993b). Such offenders can be more violent and more likely to find male victims. They are less likely to reach the courts and therefore less likely to receive treatment. Re-offending is common among sex offenders with learning disabilities (Day 1993). Day found that the majority of cases had committed more than one type of sex offence, 20% had committed both heterosexual and homosexual offences and 50% had offended against children. The offenders had experienced adverse psychosocial factors including parental violence, sexual abuse and multiple family pathology. Day differentiated between those who had committed sex offences only and those in whom the sexual offence was part of a larger context of offending behaviour, and suggested that the former were more amenable to treatment. These trends have been corroborated by Lindsay (2002). Women with learning disabilities constitute only a low percentage of referrals (Lindsey *et al.* 2004).

Various therapeutic interventions, such as individual and group therapy, have been used with sex offenders with learning disabilities. Even though they may be initially hard to engage in the assessment and treatment process, the use of simplified approaches that support the day-to-day reinforcement of treatment concepts is proving to be effective in this population (Lambrick and Glaser 2004). Better outcomes have been found with treatments that last for at least two years (Lindsey 2002). Sometimes it may be necessary to use antilibidinal agents such as cyproterone acetate to reduce the sexual drive.

Conclusion

The sexuality of people with a learning disability is clearly a complex area. Carers, statutory agencies and the legal system impact on this area of learning-disabled people's lives, which is a private area for most other individuals. It is important that any intervention is thought out carefully and implemented sensitively if these people are to feel valued.

References

Annas GJ (1981) Sterilization of the mentally retarded: a decision for the Courts. In: *The Hastings Center Report.* 11(4): 18–19.

Baxter C (1994) Sex education in the multiracial society. In: A Craft (ed.) *Practical Issues in Sexuality and Learning Disabilities.* Routledge, London.

Booth T and Booth W (1994) *Parenting Under Pressure: mothers and fathers with learning difficulties.* Open University Press, Buckingham.

Browning DH and Boatman B (1977) Incest: children at risk. *Am J Psychiatry.* 13: 69–72.

Carney T and Singer P (1986) Medical, income and property matters. In: *Ethical and Legal Issues in Guardianship Options for Intellectually Disadvantaged People.* Australian Government Publishing Service, Canberra.

Cooke LB and Sinason V (1998) Abuse of people with learning disabilities and other vulnerable adults. *Adv Psychiatr Treat.* 4: 119–25.

Craft A (ed.) (1987) *Mental Handicap and Sexuality: issues and perspectives.* Costello, Tunbridge Wells.

Craft A and Brown H (1994) Personal relationships and sexuality: the staff role. In: A Craft (ed.) *Practice Issues in Sexuality and Learning Disabilities.* Routledge, London.

Day K (1993) Crime and mental retardation: a review. In: K Howells and CR Hollin (eds) *Clinical Approaches to the Mentally Disordered Offender.* John Wiley and Sons, Chichester.

Department of Health (2001) *Valuing People: a new strategy for learning disability for the twenty-first century.* The Stationery Office, London.

Elvik SL, Berkowitz CD, Nicholas E, Lipman JL and Inkelis SH (1990) Sexual abuse in the developmentally disabled: dilemmas in diagnosis. *Child Abuse Neglect.* 14: 497–502.

Gillberg C and Geijer-Karlsson M (1983) Children born to mentally retarded mothers: a one- to twenty-one-year follow-up study of 41 cases. *Psychol Med.* 13: 891–4.

Grover S (2002) Menstrual and contraceptive management in women with an intellectual disability. *Med J Aust.* 176: 108–10.

Heshusius L (1987) Research on perceptions of sexuality by persons labelled mentally retarded. In: A Craft (ed.) *Mental Handicap and Sexuality: issues and perspectives.* Costello, Tunbridge Wells.

Lambrick F and Glaser W (2004) Sex offenders with an intellectual disability. *Sex Abuse.* **16:** 381–92.

Lindsay WR (2002) Research and literature on sex offenders with intellectual and developmental disabilities. *J Intellect Disabil Res.* **46(Suppl. 1):** 74–85.

Lindsay WR, Smith AH, Quinn K *et al.* (2004) Women with intellectual disability who have offended: characteristics and outcome. *J Intellect Disabil Res.* **48:** 580–90.

McKnorrie K (1989) Sterilisation of the mentally disabled in the English and Canadian law. *Int Comp Law Q.* **38:** 387–93.

Prosser J (1992) *Child Abuse Investigations: the families' perspective.* Parents Against Injustice (PAIN), Stansted.

Robinson SM (1987) Experiences of sex education programmes for adults who are intellectually handicapped. In: A Craft (ed.) *Mental Handicap and Sexuality: issues and perspectives.* Costello, Tunbridge Wells.

Sinason V (1993a) *Mental Handicap and the Human Condition.* Free Association Books, London.

Sinason V (1993b) The vulnerability of the handicapped child and adult. In: CJ Hobbs and JM Wynne (eds) *Child Abuse* (Clinical Paediatric Series). Balliere Tindall, London.

Sinason V (1994) Working with sexually abused individuals who have a learning disability. In: A Craft (ed.) *Practice Issues in Sexuality and Learning Disabilities.* Routledge, London.

Turk V and Brown H (1993) The sexual abuse of adults with learning disabilities: the results of a two-year incidence survey. *Ment Handicap Res.* **6:** 193–216.

Tymchuk A, Yokota A and Rahbar B (1990) Decision-making abilities of mothers with mental retardation. *Res Dev Disabil.* **11:** 97–109.

Tymchuk A and Andron L (1994) Rationale, approaches, results and resource implications of programmes to enhance parenting skills of people with learning disabilities. In: A Craft (ed.) *Practice Issues in Sexuality and Learning Disabilities.* Routledge, London.

Whitfield A (1989) The sterilisation of mentally impaired patients. In: *Medical Protection Society Annual Report.* Medical Protection Society, London.

Further reading

Craft A (ed.) (1987) *Mental Handicap and Sexuality: issues and perspectives.* Costello, Tunbridge Wells.

Craft A (ed.) (1994) *Practice Issues in Sexuality and Learning Disabilities.* Routledge, London.

Gunn MJ (1996) *Sex and Law: a brief guide for staff working with people with learning difficulties.* Family Planning Association, London.

Hollins S and Sinason V (2005) *Jenny Speaks Out.* The Royal College of Psychiatrists and Department of Psychiatry of Disability at St George's, University of London, London.

Jones K (1960) *Mental Health and Social Policy 1945–1959.* Routledge and Kegan Paul, London.

Roy M and Roy A (1988) Sterilisation for girls and women with mental handicap. Some ethical and moral considerations. *Ment Handicap.* **16:** 97–100.

Roy M, Corbett JA, Newton J and Roy A (1993) Women with a learning disability referred for sterilisation, assessment and follow-up. *J Obstet Gynaecol.* **13:** 270–75.

Roy M, Corbett JA, Newton J and Roy A (1993) Referrals of persons with a learning disability for fertility regulation. A regional survey. *J Obstet Gynaecol.* **13:** 361–4.

Roy M, Corbett JA, Newton J and Roy A (1993) Assessment of fertility regulations in persons with a learning disability – antecedents. *J Obstet Gynaecol.* **13:** 473–80.

Chapter 11

Intellectual disability and the law

Sidhartha Tewari

People with learning disabilities are a vulnerable group who are at risk of being exploited at different stages in their lives. A caring society has the responsibility to ensure that its most vulnerable members are appropriately cared for. The aim of this chapter is to look at the interface between the law and learning disabilities in England and Wales.

Terminology

Different terms are used to describe people with learning disability. Clinically the terms *mild, moderate, severe* and *profound* are used in relation to learning disabilities. These are often related to IQ scores, but attempts have been made to link them with the level of support that is required. The World Health Organization continues to use the term *mental retardation* to denote learning disability. Mild mental retardation corresponds to an IQ of 50 to 69 and a mental age of 9 to 12 years. These individuals may have had learning difficulties at school, and adults are usually able to work and maintain good social relationships and contribute to society. Moderate mental retardation corresponds to an IQ of 35 to 49 and a mental age of 6 to 9 years. There may be marked developmental delay in childhood, but most individuals can learn to develop some degree of independence in self-care and acquire adequate communications and academic skills. They are likely to require varying degrees of support in the community. People with severe mental retardation have an IQ of 20 to 34 and a mental age of 3 to 6 years, and have an ongoing need for support. People with profound mental retardation have an IQ of less than 20 and a mental age of less than 3 years. They have severe limitations with regard to self-care, continence, communication and mobility. The term *people with a learning disability* is now advocated by the Department of Health in preference to such terms as *mental handicap* and *mental retardation*.

Within the mental health legislation it is important to be aware that the definitions used are legal rather than clinical ones. Within the Mental Health Act (1983), the two terms used in relation to people with a learning disability are *mental impairment* and *severe mental impairment*.

Both terms mean 'a state of arrested or incomplete development of mind which includes significant impairment of intelligence and social functioning'. In addition, it is necessary that they are both 'associated with abnormally aggressive or seriously irresponsible conduct'. The difference between the two terms is that mental impairment does not amount to 'severe mental impairment'. Thus the distinction between the two is related to the severity of cognitive impairment and a matter for clinical judgement. If someone is to be detained on the grounds of mental impairment, then it is necessary that medical treatment is likely to alleviate or prevent deterioration in their condition. Such a condition does not apply for severe mental impairment.

The Sexual Offences Act (1956) refers to unlawful sexual intercourse with a woman who is, in the terminology used in the Act, a 'defective', and refers to indecent assault on a man who is a 'defective' (this term was originally used in the 1923 Mental Deficiency Act).

Health legislation

The Elizabethan Poor Law provided some assistance for people with learning disabilities and for other disadvantaged sections of society. However, with the growing number of unattached people drifting into towns, it became necessary to register and restrict the mobility of such people. The workhouse served this purpose to some extent, a trend that was consolidated by the creation of institutions for the care of people with mental illnesses and learning disabilities. The 1886 Idiots Act provided for residential care for people with learning disability in order to give them asylum and refuge. The 1913 Mental Deficiency Act greatly increased the number of people with mild learning disabilities (the 'feeble minded') detained in institutions. At that time it was believed that such men would be exploited or lead a life of crime if they did not live in the protective environment of an institution. Similarly, women were regarded as needing protection from sexual exploitation. The sexes were strictly segregated within institutions. The National Health Service Act of 1949 recognised the need for both training and day care for people with learning disabilities. However, it was not until the 1959 Mental Health Act and the introduction of informal admission (recommended by the 1957 Royal Commission) as opposed to compulsory detention that substantial numbers of people with learning disability were free to live in the community. The 1983 Mental Health Act further restricted the use of compulsory detention.

The Community Care Act of 1991 strengthened the move to care in the community for people with learning disabilities. The Act emphasised 'social care' and collaboration between health and local authorities and private and voluntary agencies.

Educational legislation

In the late nineteenth century, emphasis was placed on the schooling of the general population and, later, on the rights of children with learning disabilities to obtain an education. In 1876, the Elementary Education Act compelled all parents to send their children to school between the ages of 5 and 14 years, unless there was no school within two miles or the child was sick or otherwise unavoidably unable to attend. By 1899 school authorities were empowered to ascertain which children were 'defective' and thus unable to benefit from ordinary schools, but able to benefit from special classes or schools. The period of special schooling was designated from 7 to 16 years of age. This was changed by the 1944 Act, which introduced the term 'educationally subnormal' for individuals previously labelled as 'mentally defective'. It was not until 1970 that children with severe learning disabilities (who had previously been denied an education because they were regarded as ineducable) became the responsibility of education authorities under the Education (Handicapped Children) Act. The 1981 Education Act introduced the term 'special needs' and recommended integration into ordinary schools where possible.

Learning disability and the Mental Health Act

Usually patients are admitted to hospital for treatment with their explicit consent as informal patients. However, if they are unable or unwilling to give consent due to a 'mental disorder', their admission is governed by the Mental Health Act of England and Wales (1983). As this Act is due to be radically changed in the near future, we shall merely review the basic principles of the Act.

Compulsory admissions

There are basically three types of compulsory admission:

1 admission for assessment in an emergency (section 4)
2 admission for assessment (section 2)
3 admission for treatment (section 3).

An application for the patient's admission must be made by the nearest relative or an approved social worker, and must be supported by the written recommendation of a doctor and in the case of the admissions for assessment (section 2) and treatment (section 3) by the recommendation of two doctors, one of whom must have psychiatric experience and be approved.

In the case of an emergency admission (section 4), the patient cannot be kept in hospital for more than 72 hours. Following this, the patient's detention must cease or be replaced by a further period of detention for assessment or treatment.

For emergency admission and admission for assessment, it is necessary only that the medical recommendation states that the person is suffering from a mental disorder and that this is of a nature or degree that warrants detention for an assessment for a limited time in the interests of that person's own health or safety, or for the protection of others.

For admission for treatment, the nature of the mental disorder must be specified (e.g. mental illness, mental impairment, severe mental impairment or psychopathic disorder). Admissions for assessment are for 28 days and admissions for treatment are for 6 months in the first instance. The Act does not give a definition of 'mental illness', leaving this as a matter for clinical judgement. Psychopathic disorder is defined as 'a persistent disorder or disability of mind (whether or not including significant impairment of intelligence) which results in abnormally aggressive or seriously irresponsible conduct'. Individuals with mental impairment and psychopathic disorder are not liable to detention under the Mental Health Act 1983 unless it can be shown that medical treatment is likely to alleviate or prevent a deterioration of their condition.

It is important to realise that treatment can be initiated even when a person is admitted on an assessment order. The patient's consent should be obtained wherever possible, but the Act allows for treatment of a mentally disordered patient for 3 months without consent.

An informal patient who is in a hospital may be detained for 72 hours if it appears to the registered medical practitioner in charge that an application ought to be made for compulsory admission by an application to the hospital managers. A registered mental nurse or a registered nurse in mental handicap may detain an informal patient for 6 hours if it appears that the patient has a mental disorder to the degree that it is necessary for the health of the patient and the safety of others that he or she is immediately restrained from leaving the hospital and it is not practicable to secure the immediate attendance of the medical practitioner.

Guardianship

The purpose of guardianship is to enable patients to receive community care where it cannot be provided without the use of compulsory powers. The guardian is usually the social services authority but may also be an individual.

Any person subject to a guardianship order must be over 16 years of age and suffering from a mental disorder (mental illness, mental impairment, severe mental impairment or psychopathic disorder), and require guardianship in the interests of their own welfare or for the protection of others.

This order requires the person to:

- reside at a specified place
- attend at specified places and times for the purpose of medical treatment, occupation, education or training
- give access to the place where the person subject to the order is living, to any medical practitioner, approved social worker or other person specified by the guardian.

Two medical recommendations, one by a doctor approved under section 12 and the other from one with previous knowledge of the patient, are required before an approved social worker or nearest relative can make an application. Guardianship does not come into effect until the local social services authority responsible for the order accepts the order.

It is important to note that the order does not give any powers to administer medication by force, or to force the person to attend a specified place. However, if the person leaves the place where they are required to reside without the guardian's consent, they can be taken into custody and returned. Guardianship applies initially for a period of 6 months. It is renewable for a further 6 months and then for a year at a time.

Sections of the Mental Health Act that deal with criminal proceedings

While a person is awaiting trial they can be remanded to hospital for a report on their condition or for treatment. Both of these can last for 12 weeks. After assessment or treatment the person can be returned to the court to continue with the trial (section 35, remand for report; section 36, remand for treatment).

While awaiting sentence, the person can be brought to hospital for a limited time for assessment (Interim Hospital Order, section 38). This allows a proper assessment of the person's mental state to take place without a final commitment to remove the person from the judicial system. On sentencing, the court may direct the person to a hospital that has agreed to take them (Hospital Order, section 37). The hospital order is in effect similar to an admission for treatment (section 3). However, the nearest relative is not able to discharge the subject of the order from the hospital.

The Home Secretary also has powers to transfer sentenced prisoners as well as untried prisoners to hospital (section 47, transfer to hospital of convicted prisoner; section 48, transfer to hospital of untried prisoner).

Restriction order

On occasions, a Crown Court judge may – after consideration of the nature of the offence, the risk of further offences, the antecedents of the offender and with a view to protection of the public from serious harm – place a Restriction Order restricting discharge from a Hospital Order. Two doctors must examine the person and provide written reports. At least one of the two doctors must be approved and one must also give oral evidence before the court. Such powers also exist with the Home Secretary with regard to the transfer of prisoners to hospital (Restriction Directive).

Section 117: aftercare

This section of the Mental Health Act (1983) states that:

> It shall be the duty of the health authority to provide in conjunction with voluntary agencies aftercare services for any person to whom this section applies, until such time that the health authority and the local authority are satisfied that the person concerned is no longer in need of such services.

Patients detained under sections 3, 37 and 41 (i.e. a restriction order) are subject to section 117. It is the responsibility of the responsible medical officer in conjunction with the multi-disciplinary team to ensure that a care plan is formulated to meet the patient's health and social needs.

The care programme approach and the supervision register

All patients aged 16 years or over who are under the care of specialist mental health services are subject to the *care programme approach (CPA)*. This requires the allocation of a *key worker*, an assessment of health and social needs and a care plan agreed by the multi-disciplinary team. The key worker can be from either of the statutory agencies. The care programme approach is designed to provide a network of care in the community for people with severe mental illness so that they do not lose contact with the health and social services. The care programme approach can be viewed in three tiers:

1 minimal CPA
2 the CPA register (including section 117)
3 the supervision register.

The first tier applies to all patients receiving care from specialist mental health services. The second tier applies to a smaller number of patients with a severe and persistent major mental illness who fulfil certain other criteria. The third tier, namely the supervision register, was introduced from 1 April 1994 by guidance issued by the NHS Management Executive. Its purpose is to identify those people with severe mental illness who may be a serious risk to themselves or to others. It is the task of the clinical teams to judge the seriousness of the history of violence and the risk of future violence. However, all patients who are conditionally discharged from hospital under section 37/41 of the Mental Health Act 1983 should be included on the register. Inclusion on the register is designed to ensure that these patients receive intensive community support.

Supervised discharge

Supervised discharge was introduced on 1 April 1996, following the implementation of the Mental Health (Patients in the Community) Act 1995. It applies to patients who are:

- 16 years of age or over, *and*
- unrestricted, liable to be detained under section 3, 37, 47 or 48 of the Mental Health Act 1983 (including section 17 leave of absence), *and*
- suffering from mental illness, mental impairment, severe mental impairment or psychopathic disorder, *and*
- there is substantial risk of serious harm to the health or safety of the patient or the safety of other people, or the patient being seriously exploited, if the patient does not receive aftercare services under section 117 of the Act, *and*
- supervision is likely to help to ensure that the patient receives those services.

The supervised discharge must detail the requirements that are imposed on the patient. These can require the patient to reside at a specified place, to attend a specified place for medical treatment, occupation, education or training, and to allow the supervisor, or a person authorised by the supervisor, access to the place where the patient is to reside. The supervisor also has the power to convey the patient to a place where he or she is required to live or attend.

Mental Health Act Commission

The Mental Health Act Commission was introduced by the Mental Health Act 1983. Its main functions are as follows:

- to review the operation of the act by visiting, and talking to, detained patients as well as professionals and by inspecting documentation
- to monitor the Consent to Treatment provisions of the Act to ensure patient's rights are maintained an protected
- to appoint independent doctors for the purpose of providing second opinions for consent to treatment
- to keep under review the long-term treatment of detained patients
- to prepare for the Secretary of State a code of practice for doctors and other staff with regard to the admission and treatment of patients suffering from mental disorder

- to receive complaints regarding the detention and treatment of patients
- to monitor deaths of detained patients
- to report biennially to Parliament.

The Mental Health Act Commission does not have the power to discharge patients from detention.

Mental Health Review Tribunals

Mental Health Review Tribunals were introduced by the Mental Health Act 1959 and the role of the tribunal was extended by the 1983 Act. It is a judicial body that reviews the cases of compulsorily detained patients held under the Mental Health Act. The tribunal has to weigh and balance concern for the liberty of the patient with protection of the public.

The tribunal consists of three members, namely a legal member as chairman, a medical member (nearly always a psychiatrist) and a lay member (neither a doctor nor a lawyer). If the detained patient is the subject of a restriction order, the chairman must be a specially approved judge. It is one of the duties of the medical member of the tribunal to examine the detained patient and the medical notes prior to the hearing. The tribunal has the power to discharge a detained patient if it believes that the patient does not have a mental disorder, or that hospital treatment is not necessary. It can also order a delayed discharge or recommend leave of absence, transfer to another hospital or supervised discharge. In the case of restricted patients the tribunal can only order discharge, conditional discharge or delayed discharge.

Consent and capacity

Before medical treatment is given, consent must be obtained. For consent to be valid, three conditions must be satisfied.

1 It must be given by a competent person or a person lawfully appointed on behalf of that person.
2 It must be given voluntarily. There must not be any unfair pressure or influence from others.
3 It must be informed. This means that the person must be given information about the procedure relevant to the individual situation. (For the consent to be effective, the person should also be able to recount in their own words their understanding of the treatment.)

It is important to record all discussions and decisions relating to the obtaining of consent. There is a two-stage test to determine whether a person is 'competent'.

- Stage 1. Can they understand and retain information about the proposed treatment?
- Stage 2. Can they weigh up the information in order to make an informed choice?

It is important to make sure that assumptions about a person's competence to consent are not made on the basis of their diagnosis or because they belong to a particular care group.

In many people with learning disability, communication difficulties may hamper this assessment process. It is important to be clear about the steps that have been taken to give information and obtain their consent. To give valid consent a person must be capable of understanding the nature, purpose and likely effects of treatment. Furthermore, that person must be given the facts of the intended treatment such that they can make a decision without coercion. The information should be given to the person with a learning disability in the format that they can understand best.

The Mental Health Act provides the framework for people to receive treatment for a mental disorder if they are unable to consent. The situation is different in the treatment of physical disorders. Before the age of 16 years, the parents or guardians of children with learning disabilities (as with all children) give consent on their behalf. Between 16 and 18 years, the young person's consent is accepted if they are deemed to have mental capacity. However, if at 18 years of age the person with learning disability is not able to give consent due to incapacity, no one may consent on his or her behalf. It is considered good practice to involve the parents or other interested parties in the decision-making process when deciding whether a particular treatment is in the patient's best interest. For operative procedures, it may be wise to seek a second opinion as to whether a treatment is one that would be endorsed by a representative and responsible body of medical opinion.

Competence to give consent varies among individuals, and it is necessary to treat each case on its own merits. In the case of procedures such as sterilisation, which result in permanent loss of fertility, or termination of pregnancy, it may be necessary to seek a court ruling that the proposed treatment is not unlawful.

Mental Capacity Bill

The new Mental Capacity Bill is due to provide a statutory framework to empower and protect people who may be unable to make their own decisions. Thus common law principles with regard to people who do not have mental capacity are enshrined in a legal framework. Enduring powers of attorney and Court of Protection are also reformed and updated.

The five key principles of the bill are as follows.

1　A presumption of capacity – every adult has the right to make his or her own decisions, and must be assumed to have capacity to do so unless it is proved otherwise.
2　The right for individuals to be supported in making their own decisions – people must be given all appropriate help before anyone concludes that they cannot make their own decisions.
3　Individuals must retain the right to make what might be seen as eccentric or unwise decisions.
4　Best interests – anything done for or on behalf of people without capacity must be in their best interests.
5　Anything done for or on behalf of people without capacity should be the least restrictive of their basic rights or freedom.

The Bournewood case: admission to hospital of people who lack capacity

Previously, a person who lacked capacity could be detained in hospital without invoking the Mental Health Act, if they were not actively trying to leave. However, the case of H.L. (commonly referred to as the Bournewood case) is gradually changing practice with regard to hospital admission for patients without mental capacity. The case can be summarised as follows.

H.L. has autism, is unable to speak and has a limited level of understanding. He lacks the capacity to consent or object to medical treatment. After 30 years in hospital he was discharged to the community to be looked after by carers. While attending a day centre he became agitated and was admitted to hospital on an informal basis. The psychiatrist did not consider it necessary to detain H.L. under section 3 of the Mental Health Act as he was compliant, and had not resisted admission or tried to run away. His carers sought a judicial review on his behalf on the hospital's decision to admit him. The High Court rejected his application. However, the Court of Appeal (on 29 October 1997) found in favour of H.L. that he had been unlawfully detained. Although H.L. was discharged back to his carers, the case went to the House of Lords. On 25 June 1998 the House of Lords ruled by a majority that H.L. had not been detained and that he had been lawfully admitted as an informal patient on the basis of the common law doctrine of necessity. This was then taken to the European Court of Human Rights, and in 2004 the Court's seven judges unanimously held that there had been a violation with regard to both the right to liberty and security and the right to have the legality of the detention reviewed by a court.

It is likely that this judgement will lead to a shift in the use of the Mental Health Act for admission to hospital of people without mental capacity.

The Human Rights Act

The Human Rights Act 1998 came into force in October 2000. It applies to all public authorities, including NHS trusts, private and voluntary sector providers, local authorities (including social services) and the police. The Act enables people in the UK to enforce their existing European Convention rights and freedoms in the UK courts.

The 16 basic rights in the Human Rights Act are listed in Box 11.1.

Box 11.1: Rights under the Human Rights Act

Article 2	Right to Life (Article 1 is introductory)
Article 3	Prohibition of Torture
Article 4	Prohibition of Slavery
Article 5	Right to Liberty and Security
Article 6	Right to a Fair Trial
Article 7	No Punishment Without Law
Article 8	Right to Respect for Private and Family Life

Article 9	Freedom of Thought, Conscience and Religion
Article 10	Freedom of Expression
Article 11	Freedom of Assembly and Association
Article 12	Right to Marry
Article 14	Prohibition of Discrimination (Article 13 not included)
Article 1 of Protocol 1	Protection of Property
Article 2 of Protocol 1	Right to Education
Article 3 of Protocol 1	Right to Free Elections
Articles 1 and 2 of Protocol 6	Abolition of the Death Penalty

It is unclear how the Human Rights Act will affect people with learning disability. However, the Bournewood case has certainly highlighted how common law principles can be at variance with the Human Rights Act.

Declaratory relief

Everyone working in the field of adult protection should be aware of declaratory relief. The High Court can make declarations regarding the best interests of an adult who is mentally incapable of making or communicating a decision about a particular matter. Thus, in cases outside the remit of the Mental Health Act where a person does not have mental capacity, it is possible to ask the courts to make a decision regarding a serious and possibly contentious issue. It can be regarded as a form of wardship for adults. Declaratory relief is a common-law remedy that can be obtained from the Family Division of the High Court.

If doctors are unsure whether to treat or withhold treatment for a patient whose capacity or condition is such as to make informed consent unclear, the courts are sometimes asked to decide on the matter. Recently the courts have been more willing to make declarations on more general protection issues, such as where a person without competence should reside, what the arrangements for personal care should be or who has contact with that person.

Evidence is required on two issues:

1 evidence with regard to incapacity, which is usually provided by a reputable clinician who has expertise in such matters
2 evidence with regard to the best interests of the person, with clear proposals regarding daily living arrangements and reasons for their necessity.

Declaratory relief is expensive both financially and in time. The proceedings take place in a High Court and a barrister is required. Reports are required from the clinicians as well as from social workers, and both may be required to attend the court.

Sexual relationships

Under general law, 16-year-old men and women may have sexual relationships with the opposite sex. A man is said to be incapable, by law, of having sexual intercourse until he is 14 years of age, regardless of his actual biological capacity. Women may have a homosexual relationship at the age of 16 years. The law is different for men in this respect, the age of consent for homosexual acts being 18 years (this was recently lowered from 21 years by the Criminal Justice Act 1995). A man or woman can marry at the age of 16 years if they have parental consent, and at the age of 18 years without parental consent.

It is an absolute offence for a man to have sexual intercourse with a girl under the age of 13 years, and there can be no legal defence. If the girl was aged between 13 and 16 years, the man could claim in his defence that he believed that he was married to the girl or that he believed that the girl was over the age of 16 years (and that he was under the age of 24 years and had not been charged with similar offences).

According to the Sexual Offences Act of 1956, it is an offence for a man to have unlawful sexual intercourse with a woman who is a 'defective'. The term 'defective' as used to describe a person with learning disabilities is defined in the Act as a state of arrested or incomplete development of the mind which includes severe impairment of intelligence and social functioning. It is also an offence for anyone to procure a female 'defective' in order to have unlawful sexual intercourse, or for anyone to take a 'defective' away from her parents with the purpose of her having unlawful intercourse with that man. The word 'unlawful' is taken to mean 'outside the bounds of matrimony'.

Prosecutions for having sexual intercourse with someone who falls under the legal description of 'defective' are rare for a number of reasons. There is a certain amount of discretion available to the police (with regard to bringing charges) and to the Crown Prosecution service (with regard to prosecution). The guidance is that the Crown Prosecutor should take into account the ages of the participants, their relative ages, and whether there was any element of seduction or corruption in the offences before deciding whether to prosecute. Another reason is that it is extremely difficult for a layperson to judge the degree of impairment of intelligence and social functioning of someone who may be a 'defective'. Furthermore, a legal defence may be that the person was unaware (or had no reason to suspect) that the woman was a 'defective'.

The Sexual Offences Act of 1967 also deals with homosexual relationships and men with 'severe mental handicap'. All other men aged 18 years or over, except those in the armed forces, are legally able to enter into a homosexual relationship in privacy. There is no law making specific reference to relationships between women.

Other aspects of sexuality are addressed in Chapter 10.

Marriage and learning disability

People with a learning disability are often discouraged from marrying, although many wish to do so and have as much right to do so as anyone else. Both parties must be over the age of 16 years, and must understand the nature of marriage and its duties and responsibilities. They must also consent to marriage without duress.

The burden of proof regarding lack of capacity to enter a marriage rests with the person who is seeking to oppose the marriage.

Detained patients in hospital also have the right to marry, and a marriage ceremony can take place within a hospital. It is advisable for the hospital to arrange counselling for detained patients who wish to marry.

People with learning disabilities as witnesses

The learning disabled may be witnesses to crime, as they are likely to live in areas where crime is prevalent. They are also at greater risk of having a crime committed against them than the general population. Being a victim of crime can be a terrifying experience for a person without learning disability, and the existence of learning problems may make the process even more difficult. Even though a person is a victim of a crime, in the eyes of the law he or she is a witness to that crime and it is the Prosecution's brief to prepare a case against the alleged perpetrator. It is therefore important that the witness is competent and reliable. A person is judged to be a competent and reliable witness if they are able to understand the nature and sanction of the oath and to distinguish between fact and fantasy. This may be difficult for a person with learning disabilities.

There is a view that people with learning disabilities make less able witnesses because they have memory problems. However, although people with learning disabilities may provide less information overall, there is evidence that they do include the most important details. It is believed that open, free-recall questions (e.g. 'What happened?') are likely to elicit a more accurate account than closed questions (e.g. 'Was he tall?').

Gudjonsson and Clark (1986) point out that people with a learning disability are more likely to be suggestible to the answers they believe the questioner requires of them than the general population. Suggestibility is related to the memory capacity of the individual as well as to the pressures caused by the interview. There is also some evidence that people with a learning disability are more likely to say 'yes' in answer to questions that require a yes/no response, to repeated questions or to questions that they do not understand.

The prosecution, the defence, or both may request reports from expert witnesses such as psychiatrists or psychologists regarding the suggestibility of a witness. Suggestibility is difficult to quantify, and requires a detailed clinical assessment. Gudjonsson and Gunn (1982) used a method of multiple interviews, in which questions were asked in later interviews regarding facts mentioned in earlier interviews, and they also attempted to induce false perceptions or recollections of these previous interviews. For example, they would suggest that blocks shown to the person in a previous interview were black or green, whereas in fact they were red or white.

The Police and Criminal Evidence Act 1984

This Act seeks to protect vulnerable people (e.g. those with learning disabilities) during the process of interviews by the police. A person with learning disabilities must not be interviewed or asked to provide or sign a written statement without the presence of an appropriate adult.

An appropriate adult is defined in the Code of Practice as follows:

1 a relative, guardian or other person responsible for the person's care or custody
2 someone who has experience in dealing with people with learning disabilities, but is not a police officer or employed by the police (e.g. an approved social worker)
3 some other responsible adult aged 18 years or over who is not a police officer or employed by the police.

In some circumstances it may be more useful for all concerned if the appropriate adult is someone who has experience in the care of people with learning disabilities, rather than a relative who lacks such qualifications. The role of the appropriate adult is to assist the person with learning disabilities in understanding what is said to them by the police. This includes the 'caution', which must be repeated in the presence of the appropriate adult if it has already been given previously. The appropriate adult has a duty to interrupt and stop undue harassment of the suspect.

In the case of an emergency, when a delay could cause immediate harm to individuals or serious loss of or damage to property, a police officer above the rank of Superintendent may interview a person with learning disabilities without an appropriate adult being present. Questioning in these circumstances may not continue once sufficient information has been obtained to avert the immediate risk.

Fitness to plead

Fitness to plead is a question that is decided by a jury, with advice from expert witnesses such as a psychiatrist. During trials where the accused has learning disabilities, this question is often asked. To be fit to plead at the time of trial the person must:

1 understand the nature and possible consequences of the charge
2 understand the difference between a plea of guilty and a plea of not guilty
3 be able to instruct his or her lawyer
4 be able to follow the evidence in court
5 have the ability to object to a particular person becoming a juror at the trial.

Each case must be judged on its individual merits, but in general people with severe learning disabilities are unfit to plead. If the person is found not fit to plead, being 'under disability', then a 'trial of the facts' is held in the absence of the accused. The outcome of this may be that the jury find the accused either 'not guilty' or liable to be dealt with as a person under disability by admission to a treatment facility on a hospital order with or without a restriction order.

Property and people with learning disabilities

Court of Protection

Part VII of the 1983 Mental Health Act (England and Wales) governs the workings of the Court of Protection. This is an office that has powers to manage the estates of people who, because they have a mental disorder, are unable to manage their property and financial affairs. The groups of people to whom the court of protection could apply include people with severe learning disability, dementia or acquired brain damage. The Court of Protection will supervise a mentally disordered person's finances when a medical certificate supports an application. In practice, the Court of Protection is more useful when large sums of money are involved, as those who use it finance the operation of the court. In Scotland, the courts may appoint a curator bonis to manage the financial affairs of an incapacitated person.

Wills

To make a valid will (known legally as the person's testamentary capacity), the person must:

1 understand the nature and implications of making a will
2 have some appreciation of the extent of his estate
3 have some appreciation of the people who may have a reasonable expectation of being beneficiary to the estate (even though he may choose to exclude them).

There is no reason why a person with learning disabilities cannot make a valid will. Each case must be carefully examined to ensure that all the requirements are met.

Learning disability and crime

Most cultures recognise that a person with a mental disorder who breaks the law should be treated differently from a person who does not have such a disorder. Such a diversion away from a punitive sentence can result in hospitalisation.

Historically, as well as legally, the first question that is asked is about the nature of the disorder. A mental illness tends to be an acquired condition, which may be categorised into diagnostic groups. However, a learning disability:

1 is nearly always present from birth or early childhood
2 is an irreversible condition in which a person's brain does not develop as quickly or function as well as in other people
3 results in incomplete intellectual development, and in limited capacity with regard to speech, literacy, social skills and ability to learn.

Although it is realised that people with a mental disorder need to be treated differently, there has also been a strong belief that such people were more likely to commit crimes, and this resulted in their being detained in hospital or prison for longer periods of time. Such beliefs, as well as lack of suitable discharge facilities, result in long inpatient stays even today.

Very few people with severe learning disabilities are found within the criminal justice system, although many behavioural problems exhibited by those with severe or profound learning disabilities could be regarded as offences if committed by more able people. Legally it has to be shown not only that they committed the offence (actus reus), but also that they intended to commit the offence (mens rea).

There are many myths about the relationship between psychiatric disorder and crime. In the area of learning disabilities, some of the common assumptions are even less well founded. Early surveys (Goring 1913; Goddard 1920) found that much delinquency could be attributed to 'low-grade mentality', but these studies were methodologically unsound, especially with regard to the assessment of intelligence. Sutherland (1931) examined intelligence scores in the criminal population and found that they were very similar to those of the general population. East *et al.* (1942) studied 4000 juvenile offenders aged between 16 and 20 years and found that the reported IQ for the sex offenders was significantly lower than that for other offenders. Woodward (1955) concluded that low intelligence by itself played little or no part in delinquency, except in sexual offences, where there was an association. She believed that educational back-wardness was a common phenomenon among delinquents of all levels of intelligence. She also drew attention to the social and cultural factors that predispose to delinquency. These factors are also common to some people with mild learning disabilities.

In 1966, Bluglass examined 300 unselected prisoners and found that 2.6% of them had mental retardation and 11.6% had borderline intelligence. He found that the 'retarded' prisoners were more likely to be involved with property offences, to have a poor work record, to misuse alcohol and to have high levels of emotional instability. He found 'no essential difference between the distribu-tion of intelligence among convicted prisoners in general and the normal population', and was unable to find any specific association between the type of psychiatric disorder and the nature of the crime. Walker and McCabe (1973) studied 1160 offenders subject to Hospital Orders (compulsory admission to hospital for treatment), and found that one-third of them had learning disabil-ities. One-third of the men with learning disabilities accounted for 59% of the sexual offences, most of the victims being children. Among the women with learning disabilities, sexual offences tended to involve soliciting, prostitution and incest, which suggests that they may have been victims as much as offenders. People with mild learning disabilities were under-represented among the group involved in serious violent offences. This study also found an association between arson and learning disabilities. Offenders with learning disabilities (both men and women) tended to offend earlier, but their offences tended to be taken less seriously by the courts.

Various studies have examined possible associations between specific learning disability and crime. These studies have included investigations of the prevalence of aggressive and offending behaviour in men with sex chromosome abnormal-ities. Earlier studies (Jacobs *et al.* 1965; Casey *et al.* 1966) found a higher prevalence of sex chromosome abnormalities, such as 47XXY and 47XYY, in secure hospitals. It was thus postulated that these chromosomal abnormalities in some way predisposed individuals to criminal behaviour. These findings have been challenged in studies that have employed rigorous methodology, such as that by Ratcliffe (1994) in Edinburgh.

Phenotypic males with 47XXY (Klinefelter syndrome) tend to have low-normal intelligence and show an increased vulnerability to some personality disorders and other psychiatric disorders. The current view is that any link between 47XYY and criminality is tenuous. Men with additional Y chromosomes tend to be of above-average height and low-normal intelligence. It may be that their dispro-portionate presence in high-security areas reflects the response of judges to convicted offenders who are tall and have below-average intelligence.

Sexual offences

Most sex offenders do not have learning disabilities. However, sexual offences are over-represented among offences committed by people with learning disabilities. Approximately one-third to one-half of offenders with learning disabilities who are admitted to hospitals are sexual offenders (Day 1988). Most of the index offences are relatively minor, such as indecent exposure.

Sex offenders with learning disabilities tend to be characterised by psychological and social deprivation, behavioural problems at school, poor impulse control, low self-esteem and less ability to form normal sexual and personal relationships.

Sexual immaturity and lack of experience are more important aetiological considerations than sexual perversion or sexual deviancy. Often such offenders are shy, rather inept people who lack impulse control. Sometimes they are only able to relate to children, and it is in this context that they offend towards children. Many such sex offenders have themselves been victims of sexual and physical abuse in their childhood. Their victims tend to be younger children and male children.

The risk of re-offending appears to be increased if there is a long history of multiple offences, if offences were against both male and female victims, and if offences were against both children and adults.

Arson

Fire setting is over-represented among people with learning disabilities, although only a tiny proportion exhibit this behaviour. Such offenders are typically late adolescents or young adult males, often with a disrupted home background and a history of long-term behaviour problems. They tend to differ from other offenders in being generally inadequate, passive individuals, usually single, with a history of destructiveness towards property and an absence of aggression towards others (Lewis and Yarnell 1951). Often the act of setting fires may be a way of communicating their distress or anger, or an act of revenge (Jackson *et al.* 1987).

It is much rarer for women to set fires. Those who do so often have a chronic history of emotional problems, self-injury and criminal damage. There are often suspicions of sexual abuse in childhood as well as promiscuity later. Usually they have a low-normal or mild learning disability (Tennent *et al.* 1971).

Treatment facilities

Courts have a variety of options when dealing with offenders with learning disabilities. The first is a probation order with a condition that the individual attends a psychiatric outpatient clinic for treatment. Hospital treatment is indicated if:

1 the offence is serious and a custodial sentence would normally be considered
2 there is a significant risk to the public
3 there is a general need for care, training, supervision and control
4 an in-depth assessment of the person is required which cannot occur outside the hospital setting (Day 1993).

The offender may be admitted to a psychiatric or learning disability hospital under a Hospital Order (section 37) with or without restriction (section 41). Some may require secure provision for their treatment because they pose a significant risk to others or to themselves. The degree of security can range from a locked ward in a learning disability hospital to specialist low-security units, regional secure units or special hospitals. Of the three special hospitals in England, Rampton Hospital in Retford, Nottinghamshire tends to cater for people with learning disabilities. The Special Hospital Service Authority manages the special hospitals.

Treatment methods

The aims of treatment are as follows:

- to assist maturation and improve self-control
- to improve feelings of self-worth and responsibility
- to improve social, occupational and educational skills
- to address offence-specific factors (Day 1999).

General measures include life skills training which will help the person in everyday life (e.g. basic cooking, managing their money, how to find out information and obtain help). Recreation, occupation and education are also important factors in improving the person's positive self-image. Often local further education facilities can provide invaluable assistance in this context. Social skills training, often using role play, can be a very important method of improving the internal resources of a person in order to prevent re-offending. Counselling and general support are also key components of any treatment programme.

Much effort has to be made to support and involve the family in the treatment process. However, when there are dysfunctional family processes involved, measures must be taken to protect the subject and to help them to come to terms with their family's shortcomings.

Behavioural programmes are often used to link behaviour with its consequences. Various different schemes, including token economies and point schemes, have been described. Such programmes must endeavour not to be punitive but to encourage desirable behaviours.

A history of psychiatric illness is present in one-third of offenders with a learning disability, and the assessment and treatment of any illness found are clearly indicated (Day 1993). Minor physical disabilities are common, and their treatment can also help to improve self-esteem.

Medications are often used to control behaviours when there are no symptoms of mental illness, and this has resulted in some public concern, especially when these drugs are used to excess. However, in cases where brain damage is present, neuroleptics, lithium and some anti-epileptics are all effective mood stabilisers (Clarke 1997). Antilibidinal drugs are highly effective in reducing sex drive and sexual response in the learning disabled (Clarke 1989), and can be used effectively in the management of sex offenders.

Anger management training, relaxation therapy and problem solving are often used in the treatment of aggressive people. Anger management techniques seek to teach the subject how to recognise feelings of anger, and also when, where and why these feelings occur. The person is then given training in the use of self-regulatory methods to prevent angry feelings from being displayed. Training is usually undertaken in group settings, but can also be done individually.

Sex offenders with learning disability can be divided into the following three treatment groups.

1 *Developmental group.* These individuals tend to be shy and immature, and their sexual offences can be viewed as normal sexual impulses that are carried out in a crude or inept manner. This group tends to require treatments that improve their overall social skills, sexual knowledge and self-confidence, and that also improve their interpersonal and relationship skills. Antilibidinal medication and a sex behaviour management programme may be considered in this group.

2 *Antisocial group.* These individuals offend as part of a generalised antisocial behaviour disorder. They show personality disorder, psychosocial pathology and other maladaptive behaviours, and are more likely to commit serious offences and re-offend. They require both anger and sex behaviour management programmes. Antilibidinal medication and treatment in specialised treatment units are also more likely to be necessary.

3 *Sexually deviant group.* These individuals offend exclusively against children or show features of exhibitionism, cross-dressing or other fetishism. Some success has been reported as a result of using behaviour techniques in an attempt to reduce deviant sexual orientation to more normal orientation. However, sexual behaviour programmes and antilibidinal drugs are a more realistic option.

Specific treatment methods for fire setters focus on assertiveness training, instilling an understanding of the offence cycle, increasing social and communication skills, and training the individual in coping strategies such as relaxation, self-talk, avoidance and escape techniques (Day 1999).

Do treatments work?

Studies have found that about 40–70% of untreated offenders re-offend. Various different studies have found re-offending rates of between 20% and 55% following treatment, depending on the type of treatment and the offence. The risk of re-offending appears to be highest within the first year of discharge. The outcome for patients who have been treated for two years or longer appears to be more favourable and more durable than for those who have been treated for less than one year. Furthermore, good-quality aftercare following discharge improves the outcome.

Although overall rates of re-offending after treatment are high, this may be an overly pessimistic picture, as global assessments indicate a better outcome in terms of social adjustment (Day 1999).

Risk taking, risk assessment and dangerousness

Workers in the field of learning disability have a duty to protect those under their care and to prevent harm to others resulting from the behaviour problems, challenging behaviours or mental illness that their clients may have. However, they also have a duty to uphold their clients' rights as citizens. These conflicting demands mean that carers have to make decisions after balancing the risks and benefits. Taking risks and the risk of failure are part of growing up. People with learning disabilities should have the opportunity to succeed or fail at a task while learning it. Someone who has never been given the opportunity to cross a road by him- or herself can never hope to achieve road sense. However, there is a possibility of serious accident or death occurring during the process of learning, and it is on these occasions that an assessment of risk must be undertaken by staff. Another clinical example of risk assessment may be the decision-making process with regard to allowing a person with learning disability and sexual-offending behaviour unescorted leave from hospital. In this case a carefully thought out risk assessment process is required.

Risk assessment should be as thorough and objective as possible, and should examine all of the possible outcomes, ranging from desirable (positive) to undesirable (negative). The risks also have a certain likelihood or probability of occurrence. It is unlikely that a numerical value can be given to the likelihood of a particular event, but it may be helpful to assign a numerical value (e.g. 1 for certainty that an event will occur and 0 for it being impossible).

When evaluating a particular risk, a decision must be taken as to whether the objective will be of benefit to the person with learning disabilities by enhancing their independence, freedom and quality of life. No single person should have to decide on objectives and risks, but rather a team consisting of different professionals, care staff, managers, advocates and relatives is best able to take these decisions. It is extremely important from a legal point of view that the decisions, the decision-making process and the names of the people who are making the decisions are recorded in order to protect staff from future litigation.

Healthcare professionals are often expected to make predictions with regard to dangerousness in order to protect patients and others. Risk assessment here will involve knowledge of the factors that have led to the need to assess the risk to others. These will include the following:

1 any previous history of offending behaviour
2 the nature of previous and current offences
3 environmental factors
4 personality features
5 the likelihood of successful treatment
6 a history of family criminality
7 poor parenting experiences.

Among people with learning disabilities, poor self-control, low frustration tolerance and emotional detachment from the effects of offences on victims are important indicators of dangerousness. There is evidence that an offender with a record of two offences of a serious nature will commit further offences. However, this is a statistical generalisation and cannot be used to make predictions in individual cases.

It may be as well to remind ourselves that most mentally ill or learning-disabled people do not present an increased risk of violence to others.

References

Bluglass R (1966) *A psychiatric study of Scottish convicted prisoners.* MD thesis, University of St Andrews, St Andrews.
Casey MD, Blank CE, Street DRK *et al.* (1966) XYY chromosomes and antisocial behaviour. *Lancet.* **ii**: 859–60.

Clarke DJ (1989) Antilibidinal drugs and mental retardation: a review. *Med Sci Law.* **29:** 136–48.

Clarke D (1997) Physical treatment. In: SG Read (ed.) *Psychiatry in Learning Disability.* WJ Saunders, London.

Day K (1988) A hospital-based treatment programme for mentally handicapped offenders. *Br J Psychiatry.* **153:** 635–44.

Day K (1993) Crime and mental retardation: a review. In: K Howells and CR Hollin (eds) *Clinical Approaches to the Mentally Disordered Offender.* John Wiley & Sons, Chichester.

Day K (1999) Offenders with mental retardation. In: CR Hollin (ed.) *Handbook of Offender Assessment and Treatment.* John Wiley & Sons, Chichester.

East WN, Stocks P and Young HTP (1942) *The Adolescent Criminal: a medico-sociological study of 4000 male adolescents.* Churchill, London.

Goddard HH (1920) *Human Efficiency and the Levels of Intelligence.* Princeton University Press, Princeton, NJ.

Goring C (1913) *The English Convict.* HMSO, London.

Gudjonsson GH and Clarke NK (1986) Suggestibility in police interrogation: a social psychological moel. *Soc Behav.* **1:** 189-93.

Gudjonsson GH and Gunn J (1982) The competence and reliability of a witness in a criminal court: a case report. *Br J Psychiatry.* **141:** 624–7.

HMSO (1983) The Mental Health Act (1983). HMSO, London.

Jackson HF, Glass C and Hope S (1987) A functional analysis of recidivistic arson. *Br J Clin Psychol.* **26:** 175–85.

Jacobs PA, Brunton M, Melville MM, Brittain RP and McClermont WF (1965) Aggressive behaviour, mental subnormality and the XYY male. *Nature.* **208:** 1351–2.

Lewis NDC and Yarnell H (1951) *Pathological Fire Setting (Pyromania).* Nervous and Mental Disease Monograph No. 82. Coolidge Foundation, New York.

Ratcliffe (1994) The psychological and psychiatric consequences of sex chromosome abnormalities in children based on population studies. In: F Pouska (ed.) *Basic Approaches to Genetic and Molecular Biological Development Psychiatry.* Quintessenz Library of Psychiatry, Berlin.

Sutherland EH (1931) Mental deficiency and crime. In: K Young (ed.) *Social Attitudes.* Henry Holt, New York.

Tennent G, McQuaid A and Looughane T (1971) Female arsonists. *Br J Psychiatry.* **119:** 497–502.

Walker N and McCabe S (1973) *Crime and Insanity in England. Volume 2. New solutions and new problems.* Edinburgh University Press, Edinburgh.

Woodward M (1955) The role of low intelligence in delinquency. *Br J Delinquency.* **5:** 281–303.

Further reading

Ashton G and Ward A (1992) *Mental Handicap and the Law.* Sweet & Maxwell, London.

Bluglass RA (1983) *A Guide to the Mental Health Act.* Churchill Livingstone, Edinburgh.

Bluglass RA and Bowden P (eds) (1990) *Principles and Practice of Forensic Psychiatry.* Churchill Livingstone, Edinburgh.

Chiswick D and Cope R (eds) (1995) *Practical Forensic Psychiatry.* Royal College of Psychiatrists, London.

Gunn MJ (1996) *Sex and Law* (3e). Underhill, London.

Hollin CR (1999) *Handbook of Offender Assessment and Treatment.* John Wiley & Sons, Chichester.

Johnstone EC, Cunningham Owens DG, Lawrie SM, *et al.* (eds) (2004) *Companion to Psychiatric Studies* (7e). Churchill Livingstone, Edinburgh.

Jones R (1999) *Mental Health Act Manual.* Sweet & Maxwell, London.

The Maudsley Hospital (1997) *The Maze: Mental Health Act 1983. Guidelines.* Sponsored by Smith, Kline & Beecham.

Part 3

Meeting the need

This section focuses on the use of drugs in psychiatric disorder, as well as on multi-disciplinary and multi-professional working. The final section provides an outline of integrated services as informed by recent government guidance

Chapter 12

The use of psychotropic drugs in people with intellectual disabilities

Shoumitro Deb

Introduction

Psychotropic medication includes drugs such as antipsychotics, antidepressants, mood stabilisers, psychostimulants, anti-anxiety drugs and hypnotics. Some would include anti-epileptic drugs in this group. These drugs act on the central nervous system and can be used to modify human behaviour and treat psychiatric disorders, including psychological symptoms. Drugs such as beta-blockers and opioid antagonists that have an effect on human behaviour can also be regarded as psychotropic medication in this context. A high proportion of adults who have learning disabilities receive psychotropic drugs, many are on more than one drug, and many receive these drugs at a much higher dose than is recommended in the *British National Formulary* (Deb and Fraser 1994). Although these drugs are used to treat psychiatric disorders, there are also many cases where they are used to treat behaviour disorders (in the absence of a diagnosed psychiatric disorder) for which they are not indicated. For example, Clarke *et al.* (1990) showed that 36% of adults with learning disability who did not have a diagnosis of psychiatric illness also received psychotropic medication. The use of psychotropic drugs in the management of behaviour disorders *per se* in people with learning disabilities in the absence of a diagnosable psychiatric illness remains controversial (Reiss and Aman 1998; Santosh and Baird 1999; Aman *et al.* 2000; Deb and Weston 2000).

One of the reasons for such a high rate of use of psychotropics among adults with learning disabilities is the high prevalence of behaviour disorders in this population. Deb *et al.* (2001a) found a similar rate of functional psychiatric illness, such as schizophrenia, affective disorders and anxiety-related disorder, among adults with learning disabilities to that in the general population. However, the rate of behaviour disorder among adults with learning disabilities was found to be high (Deb *et al.* 2001b). The rate of psychosis is significantly higher among adults with learning disabilities compared with the general population. Other psychiatric diagnoses, such as autistic spectrum disorders and attention deficit hyperactivity disorders, which are not commonly diagnosed among the general adult population seem to be not uncommon among adults with learning disabilities. Personality disorder, although a controversial diagnosis, seems to be diagnosed by some at a higher rate among adults with learning disabilities. Therefore the overall rate of psychopathology among adults with learning disabilities seems to be much higher than that in the general population (Deb *et al.* 2001c). Furthermore, the rate of epilepsy is much higher among adults with learning disabilities than in the general population (Deb 2000). Because of all these findings, the rate of use of psychotropic medication in adults with learning disabilities is much higher than that in the general population.

Psychiatric illness

Indications for drugs for the treatment of psychiatric disorders such as psychoses (e.g. schizophrenia, schizo-affective disorder, delusional disorders), affective disorders (e.g. depressive episodes, bipolar disorders) and anxiety-related disorders (e.g. generalised anxiety disorder, obsessive-compulsive disorder, panic disorder, phobia) should be the same among people with learning disabilities as they are for the general population. Therefore in this chapter we shall discuss primarily the indications for psychotropic drugs for the treatment of behaviour disorders *per se*.

Management of behaviour disorders

The types of behaviour disorders among people with learning disabilities that usually need drug treatment include aggression towards others, aggression towards property and objects (destructiveness), aggression towards self (self-injurious behaviour, SIB), severe agitation/hyperactivity, severe stereotyped behaviour and severe temper tantrums (including screaming). At the outset it is important to assess carefully the possible cause(s) of behaviour disorders. A person with learning disabilities who is in pain but is unable to communicate this to their carer may behave in an aggressive manner out of frustration. It is therefore important to assess the individual's physical state carefully and provide the necessary treatment that might subsequently help to improve the associated behaviour disorder. Certain behaviour disorders may be the manifestation of an underlying psychiatric syndrome, such as psychoses or depression. It is therefore necessary to carefully assess the individual for an underlying psychopathology. Psychological factors such as stress and learned dysfunctional coping strategies could predispose, precipitate and perpetuate behaviour disorders. These factors need to be identified and treated with appropriate therapies. Behavioural management therapy and psychological therapies such as cognitive behavioural therapy could be useful in the management of behaviour disorders. Certain social factors, such as under- or over-stimulation within the immediate environment, physical and psychological abuse, life events and lack of social support, could predispose people with a learning disability to behaviour disorders. Thus in many cases addressing the appropriate social issues along with certain environmental manipulation may be all that is needed to manage behaviour disorders. A lack of careful assessment of the above factors may lead to unnecessary prescribing of drugs.

It is important to remember that drug treatment is one of many strategies that could be employed to manage psychopathology, and particularly behaviour disorders in people with learning disabilities. Treatment should be provided within the context of a carefully drawn up individualised care programme after proper discussion with the person with learning disabilities, their carers, and other professionals involved in the care of the person. The treatment plan should also comply with the national legal framework. The overall aim of the treatment should be not only to control symptoms but also to provide better quality of life for people with learning disabilities and to lessen their carer's burden. The treatment must also be based on the proper evidence of effectiveness of a particular treatment. Clinicians in the UK are increasingly asked to abide by the National Institute for Clinical Excellence (NICE) guidelines (www.nice. org.uk), which are primarily based on type I and type II evidence but not on case reports or expert opinions. Type I evidence includes a good systematic review and meta-analysis, including at least one randomised controlled trial. Type II evidence includes randomised controlled trials, type III evidence includes well-designed interventional studies without randomisation, type IV evidence includes well-designed observational studies, and type V evidence includes expert opinion, influential reports and studies. Unfortunately, until now we have mostly been limited to type IV and type V evidence for the effectiveness of psychotropics in the management of behaviour disorders among adults with learning disabilities.

Antipsychotics

Among typical antipsychotics, chlorpromazine, haloperidol and thioridazine are the most widely used drugs for the management of behaviour disorders in adults with learning disability. However, the use of thioridazine is now severely restricted in the UK because of its potential cardiotoxicity. Most studies, particularly in the form of case reports, have reported an improvement in the target behaviour after treatment. Atypical antipsychotics include clozapine, risperidone, olanzapine, amisulpride and quetiapine. Compared with the typical antipsychotics, atypicals have less propensity to cause extrapyramidal side-effects, and they work on a 5 hydroxy tryptamine (HT)-neuroreceptor system. Atypical antipsychotics are known to cause weight gain, diabetes, hyperprolactinaemia and QTc prolongation in the ECG. Clozapine can cause fatal blood dyscrasias in around 1% of cases, and it is therefore necessary to regularly monitor blood tests for patients who are being treated with this drug. Most studies to date have concentrated on the efficacy of risperidone. In total there are about 32 reports of the use of risperidone in the treatment of behaviour disorders among children and adults with learning disability, and among children and adults with pervasive developmental disability including autism. There are a few reports of the use of clozapine and olanzapine among people with learning disability. One or two reports have shown improvement of aggression in patients with schizophrenia when they were treated with either clozapine or quetiapine. Most studies have reported improvements following treatment with these atypical antipsychotics. However, these were mainly case reports, so no control group was used and patients were not randomised into different treatment groups. It is therefore difficult to draw any valid conclusions from these studies.

Antidepressants

Among antidepressants, most studies have reported the use of clomipramine and selective serotonin reuptake inhibitors (SSRIs) in the management of behaviour disorders among adults with learning disabilities. As these drugs are known to improve symptoms of depression, anxiety and obsessive behaviour, it is possible that the improvement in behaviour disorder in fact reflected an improvement in the above symptoms. SSRIs have been shown to be particularly effective in case studies of self-injurious behaviours. It is possible that these drugs are treating the underlying tendency toward obsessional behaviour in such cases. The severe withdrawal effects that may be caused by the stopping of SSRIs are likely to restrict their long-term use.

Mood stabilisers

Mood stabilisers are used as prophylaxis for bipolar affective disorders. These include lithium and anti-epileptic drugs such as carbamazepine, sodium valproate and lamotrigine. Almost all studies in which lithium was used to treat behaviour disorders among adults with learning disabilities showed an improvement. Blood levels of lithium should be monitored regularly initially to stabilise the level between 0.4 and 0.8 mmol/L. A higher serum level of lithium (over 1.2 mmol/L) is likely to cause lithium toxicity. Cardiac, thyroid and renal functions should also be monitored regularly in patients who are being treated with lithium. Around 88% of patients treated with valproate showed an improvement in aggression and self-injurious behaviour. Both lamotrigine and sodium valproate can cause skin rash. There are no reports on the effectiveness of lamotrigine for the treatment of behaviour disorders in adults with learning disabilities. There is a complex relationship between epilepsy and behaviour disorders in some people with learning disabilities (Deb and Joyce 1999). It is therefore possible that sodium valproate may be treating the underlying epileptic activity while showing an improvement in behaviour disorder.

Anti-anxiety drugs

Case reports have shown that both benzodiazepines and buspirone improve behaviour disorders in people with learning disabilities. There have been three randomised controlled trials involving a total of 29 patients and 16 open-label trials involving a total of 60 patients on the use of beta-blockers in the treatment of behaviour disorders in people with learning disabilities. Benzodiazepines, buspirone and beta-blockers all have an anti-anxiety effect. Anxiety could be a precipitating factor for behaviour disorders in people with learning disabilities. It is therefore possible that the above drugs produce an improvement in behaviour by treating the underlying anxiety. The long-term use of benzodiazepines is contraindicated because of the problems with tolerance, alcohol intolerance, a possible effect on cognition and symptoms associated with withdrawal. After the initial enthusiasm with regard to buspirone, recent studies have shown that it has a slow onset of action and lower potency. High-dose beta-blockers that are used for the treatment of behaviour disorders can cause cardiac problems.

Opioid antagonists

Some researchers have postulated that self-injurious behaviour is sustained by the release of internal opioids in the body. This consequently produces a feeling of pleasure, which tends to perpetuate the behaviour. Therefore the use of anti-opioid drugs such as naloxene and naltrexone has been proposed for the treatment of self-injurious behaviour in people with learning disabilities. However, to date the efficacy of naloxene and naltrexone has not been unequivocally demonstrated in the management of self-injurious behaviour in people with learning disabilities.

Psychostimulants

Psychostimulants such as methylphenidate and dexamphetamine have been successfully used in conjunction with behavioural and psychological treatments in the management of attention deficit hyperactivity disorder (ADHD) in children. Some case reports have demonstrated the successful use of these drugs in the treatment of behaviour disorders in people with learning disabilities. However, many adults with learning disabilities show symptoms of ADHD that could be associated with behaviour disorders. It is therefore possible that psychostimulants produce an improvement in behaviour disorders by treating the underlying ADHD symptoms. To date the effects of long-term use of psychostimulants and their eventual withdrawal have not been properly studied.

Other drugs

Clonidine, which is an anti-hypertensive drug, is also indicated for the treatment of tic disorder and Tourette's syndrome. There have been studies of the use of clonidine in the treatment of behaviour disorders in people with learning disabilities. Both tic disorder and Tourette's syndrome are known to be associated with learning disability and behaviour disorders. Vitamins, minerals and dietary treatments (particularly in patients with phenylketonuria) have also been used with some success in the treatment of behaviour disorders in people with learning disabilities.

Quality of the evidence

It is clear from the evidence presented here that many studies have shown the effectiveness of psychotropic drugs in the treatment of behaviour disorders in adults with learning disability. However, we must be cautious when interpreting the data presented in these studies. Most of these studies are case reports that included a small number of cases. It is well known that studies with positive findings tend to find their way to publication more easily than studies that show negative findings, which creates a reporting bias. The number of randomised controlled trials is small, and they often used a small cohort size, so they have insufficient statistical power to allow firm conclusions to be drawn. The outcome measures used in these studies are often not appropriate or validated. The method of selection of control and experimental groups is not always clear or appropriate. Furthermore, outcome data are often not presented in an appropriate manner. For example, most studies do not report the 'number needed to treat' or use analysis based on 'intention to treat'. Most studies also did not distinguish between symptoms of psychiatric illness and those of behaviour disorders. Often researchers did not take into account the existence of autistic and ADHD symptoms in the context of behaviour disorders. It therefore remains unclear whether the drugs used in these studies treated the underlying psychiatric condition or the behaviour disorder *per se*. Although there is no strong evidence to suggest the effectiveness of psychotropic drugs in the management of behaviour disorders in adults with learning disabilities, there is also no strong evidence that these drugs are ineffective. Properly controlled randomised studies are needed to answer the question of whether or not psychotropic drugs are effective, and at present such studies are simply not available.

A systematic review conducted by Brylewski and Duggan (2004) for the Cochrane Review group highlighted most of the methodological problems that I have listed above. By using strict criteria for the inclusion of randomised controlled trials they found only six studies that provided sufficient information or used appropriate methodology and so qualified for inclusion in their review. They found no evidence either way to suggest that drugs are either useful or not useful in the treatment of behaviour disorders in people with learning disability.

ADHD and autistic spectrum disorders

Psychostimulants such as methylphenidate in association with other methods of behaviour management have been shown to be effective in the treatment of ADHD. There is an association between ADHD and learning disability. Psychostimulants have been shown to be equally effective in the treatment of ADHD in children with learning disabilities. Many reports have shown the effectiveness of different drugs in the treatment of core symptoms and associated behaviour disorders in children with autistic spectrum disorders. The quality of evidence is often poor and unreliable, but it is possible that the same indications for drug treatment should apply to children with autism in the presence of learning disability. Santosh and Baird (1999) suggested the use of methylphenidate or clomipramine for hyperactivity, SSRIs for self-injurious behaviour, haloperidol, risperidone, buspirone or clonidine for irritability and aggression, and clonazepam, buspirone or beta-blockers for anxiety symptoms in children with autistic spectrum disorders. They also recommended the use of haloperidol, risperidone, sulpiride, clonidine, SSRIs, clomipramine or a combination of these drugs in the treatment of tic disorder/Tourette's syndrome. They suggested the use of clonidine for hyperactivity, aggression or hyperarousal, and tricyclics or buspirone for children with combined symptoms of autism and ADHD. However, the suggestions of Santosh and Baird (1999) are based on anecdotes and expert opinions rather than on any hard evidence.

Scope for drug withdrawal

Many people with learning disabilities receive psychotropic drugs for many years without any proper assessment of their treatment. Ahmed *et al.* (2000) and Branford (1996) conducted important studies to assess which factors affect the withdrawal of long-term use of these drugs. Ahmed *et al.* (2000) successfully reduced the dose of antipsychotic medication without the resurgence of behaviour disorders in 52% of a sample of 36 adults with learning disabilities, of whom 33% completed the full withdrawal programme. These researchers found that not only an individual's behaviour but also factors such as staff perception, environmental factors, staffing ratios and administrative and treatment philosophies influenced prescribing habits.

Practice guideline

In the absence of unequivocal evidence to support the use of psychotropic medication for the treatment of behaviour disorders among people with learning disabilities, it is important to follow certain practice guidelines, which should provide clinicians with a framework for the use of these drugs. Clinicians who are prescribing drugs for people with learning disabilities also need to be aware of issues relating to capacity, informed consent, advocacy, the Mental Health Act and relevant Government documents such as *Valuing People* (www.doh.gov.uk) and *Same as You*. Practice guidelines that have been proposed by an international consensus group (Reiss and Aman 1998) are summarised in Boxes 12.1 and 12.2.

Box 12.1: Dos

- Use psychotropic medications within a coordinated multi-disciplinary care plan.
- The types of psychotropic drug that are used should be based on adequate evidence for their effectiveness.
- Use psychotropic medication based on a psychiatric diagnosis or a specific behavioural–pharmacological hypothesis, and only after conducting a complete diagnostic and functional assessment.
- Assess capacity and obtain informed consent from the individual or a carer, and establish a therapeutic alliance involving all decision makers.
- Monitor the efficacy of treatment by defining objective index behaviours and quality-of-life outcomes, and measure them using empirical methods.
- Monitor for adverse drug effects using standardised assessment instruments.
- Conduct clinical and data reviews on a regular basis and in a systematic way.
- Strive to use the lowest optimal effective dose and where possible withdrawal of drugs when indicated.
- Evaluate drug and monitoring practices through a peer or team quality review or improvement group.

Box 12.2: Don'ts

- Don't use psychotropic drugs excessively, for convenience, as a substitute for meaningful psychosocial services, or in quantities that interfere with quality of life.
- Avoid frequent drug and dose changes.
- Avoid intra-class polypharmacy and minimise inter-class polypharmacy as far as possible in order to decrease the likelihood of patient non-compliance and drug adverse effects.
- Avoid the use of high-dose antipsychotics.
- Avoid the long-term use of benzodiazepines.
- Avoid the long-term use of anticholinergic drugs.
- Avoid the long-term use of PRN ('as required') instructions.

References

Ahmed Z, Fraser W, Kerr MP *et al.* (2000) Reducing antipsychotic medication in people with a learning disability. *Br J Psychiatry.* **178:** 42–6.

Aman MG, Alvarez N, Benefield W *et al.* (2000) Expert consensus guidelines for the treatment of psychiatric and behavioral problems in mental retardation. *Am J Ment Retard.* **105:** 159–228.

Branford D (1996) Factors associated with the successful or unsuccessful withdrawal of antipsychotic drug therapy prescribed for people with learning disabilities. *J Intellect Disabil Res.* **40:** 322–9.

Brylewski J and Duggan L (2004) Antipsychotic medication for challenging behaviour in people with intellectual disability: a systematic review of randomised controlled trials. *J Intellect Disabil Res.* **43:** 360–71.

Clarke DJ, Kelley S, Thinn K and Corbett JA (1990) Psychotropic drugs and mental retardation. I. Disabilities and the prescription of drugs for behaviour and for epilepsy in three residential settings. *J Ment Defic Res.* **34:** 385–95.

Deb S (2000) Epidemiology and treatment of epilepsy in patients who are mentally retarded. *CNS Drugs.* **13:** 117–28.

Deb S and Fraser W (1994) The use of psychotropic medication in people with learning disability: towards rational prescribing. *Hum Psychopharmacol.* **9:** 259–72.

Deb S and Joyce J (1999) Psychiatric illness and behavioural problems in adults with learning disability and epilepsy. *Behav Neurol.* **11:** 125–9.

Deb S and Weston SN (2000) Psychiatric illness and mental retardation. *Curr Opin Psychiatry.* **13:** 497–505.

Deb S, Thomas M and Bright C (2001a) Mental disorder in adults with intellectual disability. I. Prevalence of functional psychiatric illness among a community-based population aged between 16 and 64 years. *J Intellect Disabil Res.* **45:** 495–505.

Deb S, Thomas M and Bright C (2001b) Mental disorder in adults with intellectual disability. II. The rate of behaviour disorders among a community-based population aged 16 and 64 years. *J Intellect Disabil Res.* **45:** 506–14.

Deb S, Matthews T, Holt G and Bouras N (eds) (2001c) *Practice Guidelines for the Assessment and Diagnosis of Mental Health Problems in Adults who have Intellectual Disability.* European Association for Mental Health in Mental Retardation (EAMHMR) in association with Pavilion Press, London.

Reiss S and Aman MG (1998) *The International Consensus Handbook: psychotropic medications and developmental disabilities.* American Association on Mental Retardation, Washington, DC.

Santosh PJ and Baird G (1999) Psychopharmacology in children and adults with intellectual disability. *Lancet.* **354:** 231–40.

Chapter 13

Professional roles and multi-disciplinary working in intellectual disability services

Meera Roy

Introduction

People with learning disabilities have a higher than average need for healthcare services. Over 60% of people in this group who live in the community have at least one chronic disorder that is sufficient to warrant ongoing medical intervention. People with a severe learning disability often have associated physical problems such as epilepsy, sensory impairment, cerebral palsy and difficulties in speech and communication. Various studies have shown that up to one-third of children with severe learning disability suffer from epilepsy. Mental health problems are three to four times more common in this group than in the general population.

Most people with learning disabilities live in the community, either with their families or with paid carers. In order to do so, they need access to a daytime occupation and opportunities for education, leisure and employment, respite care to give their families a break, and residential care in the event that their families are no longer able to look after them. The emphasis on closure of long-stay hospitals for people with learning disability has meant that they live and receive care in the community. In view of the complex needs of these people, the skills of a variety of professionals are needed. In most parts of the country these professionals work together as a team. One of the most important resources for a person with learning disability and their carers in the community is the *community learning disability team*.

Community learning disability team

Community learning disability teams usually consist of community nurses for people with learning disabilities and specialist social workers and other professionals such as psychiatrists, psychologists, occupational therapists, physiotherapists, behaviour specialists, dietitians and speech and language therapists. The team members work closely together to provide comprehensive assessments and management strategies for the people referred to the team. The philosophy of the teams is to support people with learning disabilities and their carers so as to enable them to have as ordinary and fulfilling a lifestyle as possible. As teams can be organised in different ways, it is useful to have an understanding of the specific skills of the different professionals in learning disability services.

Community nurse for people with learning disabilities

Community nurses have special training in learning disability and usually are registered nurses in learning disability (RNLD). They work in partnership with individuals to improve their autonomy by reducing the effects of disability and achieving optimum health. They facilitate and encourage involvement in local communities and maximise their clients' choice. They also enhance the contribution of others who are involved. They have a central role in health surveillance and health promotion. The White Paper, *Valuing People: a new strategy for learning disability for the twenty-first century* (Department of Health 2001) has recommended that health facilitators be appointed to improve the access of people with learning disabilities to health services. The community nurses have made this role their own, and together with the person with learning disability they draw up Health Action Plans to encourage healthy lifestyles. This may be seen as their role in primary care.

In addition, community nurses take on a specialist role in any or all of the following areas, where they can also specialise to the level of a nurse specialist:

- management of epilepsy
- monitoring and management of mental health
- providing services for older people with a learning disability
- supporting people with autistic disorders
- working with children with learning disability and their families to reduce behavioural difficulties, manage sleep problems, implement special diets and carry out systemic interventions
- implementing behavioural programmes
- managing the sequelae of severe physical disabilities such as pressure sores and peg (parenteral gastrostomy) feeding
- supporting parents with a learning disability
- bereavement counselling, anger and anxiety management, stress management and giving advice on relationship difficulties
- working with the criminal justice system to manage people with learning disabilities who offend
- managing the transition between services (e.g. children to adults' services or adults to older adults' services) so that the process is a smooth one
- working with children and adults who may have been abused.

In their role of monitoring and supporting people with learning disabilities who have psychiatric disorders, they may be care co-ordinators and supervisors for people on the care programme approach and supervised discharge (section 25 of the Mental Health Act 1983). Together with their social work colleagues, they also draw up care plans for individuals who require specialised packages of care in order to obtain funding from relevant authorities.

Nurses who work in inpatient settings have skills in many of the areas described above. In addition, they provide a stable and consistent environment in which assessments and interventions can take place.

Social worker

The primary aim of the social worker is to support, advise and assist people with a learning disability and their families in living within the local community. They provide advice on welfare benefits, housing, health and hygiene and counselling. They are also able to obtain respite care, which may be in variety of settings ranging from fostering to day care. They have a key role in protecting children and adults with a learning disability who may be at risk of being abused.

One of the main pieces of legislation with which the community teams work is the Community Care Act 1993. This entitles a person to an assessment of needs, which could be either simple or complex. An example of a simple need would be to arrange respite care for a person with a learning disability. An example of a complex need would be to find a home for a person with a learning disability who had an additional mental illness and deafness. Increasingly, teams are working with people with complex needs, which requires planning meetings and the setting up of care packages with multi-agency and multi-disciplinary input (e.g. involving psychiatrists, psychologists, and voluntary and independent agencies). The social worker is often the only individual with the responsibility for applying for funding and for monitoring and reviewing care packages.

In addition, the social worker has responsibility for people with learning disabilities who may be detained under sections of the Mental Health Act. Some obtain further training to become approved social workers, and are then able to make applications for assessment under the Act. They work closely with assessment and treatment units to formulate care plans under section 117 for people who are discharged from orders of the Mental Health Act 1983. On occasions when the nearest relative is displaced by the County Court, the approved social worker becomes the nearest relative on behalf of the local authority. When a person with a learning disability is received into guardianship under the Mental Health Act, the social worker again has a key role in monitoring the care package.

Under the Children's Act, the social worker in the children with disabilities team may also have to arrange for a child to be taken into care if the parents are no longer able to discharge their parental duties.

Occupational therapist

The primary aim of the occupational therapist is to promote and restore health and well-being in people of all ages using purposeful occupation as the process or the ultimate goal. In this context, occupation is the meaningful use of activities, occupations, skills and life roles, which enables people to function purposefully in their daily life.

The occupational therapist adopts a holistic, client-centred approach that is shaped by the principles of social role valorisation. This is useful for providing a framework within which individual needs can be assessed where appropriate and therapeutic programmes of intervention can be devised to maximise levels of functioning and independence. Assessments take place in a variety of settings (e.g. the client's home and day centres) and involve both clients and their families. The occupational therapist obtains a relevant medical and social history as well as details of life events and current life roles. Criterion-based assessment (e.g. star profile), occupational therapy checklists and task analysis of activities are carried out. At the end of this process, a planned programme of intervention is devised.

Occupational therapists enable people with learning disabilities to maximise their physical, emotional, cognitive and functional potential by teaching them or enhancing skills such as eating, dressing, cooking and shopping. The skills necessary for the above activities can be improved by memory training and improving physical ability. The therapists help clients to prepare for more independent living and manage anxiety. They adapt techniques to maintain independence (e.g. using pictorial checklists for cleaning routines and shopping lists). Group work techniques encourage social interaction. The home environment can be manipulated to increase independence or to enhance quality of life by providing specialised equipment such as bath aids, eating utensils and adaptations to compensate for dysfunction (e.g. improving accessibility for wheelchair users).

In recent years, occupational therapists have been involved in carrying out assessments of how people on the autistic spectrum process sensory information. As was described in Chapter 4, people with autistic conditions have unusual sensory processing, as a result of which they are either hyper- or hyposensitive to different stimuli. Occupational therapists are able to identify stimuli that cause distress, challenging behaviours which can be avoided, and pleasurable ones which can then be incorporated into a sensory diet to facilitate relaxation. Access to an occupational therapist who is able to carry out such an assessment would reduce the need for psychotropic medication in these people.

Occupational therapists enable clients to have a meaningful lifestyle by appropriate use of leisure, exploring opportunities for education and training, and achieving a balance between personal, domestic, leisure and education/work-related activities. They also provide practical advice for clients and carers to maintain independence where deterioration in ability is anticipated (e.g. in individuals with a progressive neurological deficit).

Clinical psychologist

The clinical psychologist within the multi-disciplinary team works with clients who have problems that are considered to be amenable to psychological intervention. In addition to direct client work, the psychologist can offer support and supervision to colleagues who have adopted a psychological approach to their work. Clinical psychologists who work with people with learning disability use a range of psychological models, including the cognitive behavioural approach, the humanistic approach to therapy, psychodynamic approaches and behavioural approaches to treatment.

Clinical psychology is the application of psychological theory and research when working with people to promote health and to cure and prevent illness. Psychological approaches can be applied to a range of difficulties, including relationship problems, sexual dysfunction, depression, anxiety, obsessive-compulsive disorders, eating disorders, alcohol-related problems and conduct disorders. Psychological techniques have also been applied to a range of lifestyle issues, such as stress inoculation, smoking cessation and weight reduction.

Behavioural approaches have moved from 'modification techniques', which were often punitive, towards non-punitive interventions based on an analysis of the problem situations. It has also been recognised that the 'challenging environments' (McGill and Toogood 1994) in which clients often live can combine with their disabilities to give them no alternative 'non-challenging' ways of meeting important everyday needs (Mansell 1994). Functional analysis involves identifying the function or purpose of behaviours, the stimuli that elicit them, and the full range of individual and environmental factors that maintain or mediate the situation. The behaviour may, for example, serve a communicative function. Head banging may be the first response to headache or toothache in an individual with poorly developed communication skills. Interventions are behaviour-decreasing programmes, and can be a combination of increasing functional skills relevant to the problem, adaptation to the individual's environment (e.g. change in activities) and an emphasis on lifestyle or quality-of-life changes both as a means and an end. Clinical psychologists are often the coordinators of behaviour support teams, where they work with nurses to deliver an intensive service.

Clinical psychologists also often take a lead in working with people with learning disabilities who have been abused. As they are able to identify an individual's profile of ability, they have an important role in the assessment of capacity in relation to giving consent, whether it be for treatment or in legal proceedings. Those with skills in the area of systemic therapy have an important role in reducing behaviour difficulties, particularly in the residential setting.

Speech and language therapist

The speech and language therapist is the team expert in the area of communication abilities. The therapist obtains information about the client's communication skills, including their level of comprehension, means of expression, attention and listening skills, interaction and social skills, from informal observations and the use of formal assessments. He or she is also involved with the assessment of associated behaviour problems and feeding and drinking skills. This assessment is usually conducted over a period of time.

Interventions may be direct or indirect, and clients may be seen either individually or as part of a group. Direct intervention may, for example, be focusing on the teaching of new Makaton signs (a communication system based on British sign anguage), whereas indirect intervention would focus on transferring this skill into the everyday environment. In general, a total communication approach is advocated and includes the use of signs, symbols, objects and pictures with speech in order to maximise the communication environment and thus the communication potential of the client.

Speech and language therapists train staff, carers, parents and others involved with the learning-disabled person, and address general communication issues or train in specific skill areas (e.g. Makaton training). Training is seen both as an essential part of the overall management and as a way of encouraging successful communication within the everyday environment. The role of the speech and language therapist is most effective when the therapist is part of the multi-disciplinary team.

Physiotherapist

The physiotherapist is an expert on the assessment and analysis of movement and function. They put together individually tailored intervention programmes, incorporated where possible into everyday activities in order to provide stimulation and motivation and enable clients to gain new skills and further independence.

The purpose of the assessment is to identify strengths and weaknesses in the individual's physical development, which may include variations in muscle tone, the absence or presence of movement and the extent of physical deformities (if any). The intervention programmes may include any of the following:

- the use of sensory input to facilitate or inhibit the central nervous system
- the application of neurodevelopmental concepts
- the application of skilful manual techniques
- some principles of conductive education (hydrotherapy, swimming, education)
- the training of carers and staff in moving and handling techniques
- support for carers in their unique role, and alternatives to aggressive and challenging behaviour in the form of physical activities and exercise.

People with profound multiple handicaps are highly prone to physical deformities and increasing stiffness as they get older. The provision of several positions that are comfortable for such clients is an essential part of a daily care package. People with cerebral palsy often need intensive input from physiotherapists to maximise their functioning and reduce deterioration (characterised by contractures and reduced strength and movement). The maintenance of systematic records of people's physical abilities is useful in their long-term management.

Physiotherapists also have a key role in health promotion, and have taken the lead in introducing safe moving and handling techniques for both carers and staff, thus helping to prevent back injuries when caring for people with multiple disabilities.

Dietitian

It is important for people with learning disabilities to have access to dietitians. They are often overweight compared with the general population, partly as a result of underlying syndromes such as Prader–Willi syndrome, fewer opportunities for physical activity, a sedentary lifestyle, prescribed medication and the use of food as a source of comfort. Weight reduction is a key target in the Coronary Heart Disease National Service Framework, and dietitians have an important role to play.

Autistic disorders are more common in people with a learning disability, and people on the autistic spectrum often have food fads and preferences for certain textures. Input from the dietitian is crucial in ensuring that they have an adequate diet. People with multiple disabilities have feeding problems and difficulties in swallowing, and may need their food thickening or feeding through a gastric peg. Dietitians, speech and language therapists and physiotherapists work together to manage these complex cases.

People with learning disabilities sometimes need special diets (e.g. phenylalanine-free diets for phenylketonuria, gluten- and/or lactose-free diets for people with autism). These individuals need input from the dietitian to ensure that they have balanced meals.

Pharmacist

Pharmacists with a special interest in people with a learning disability are a valuable resource for any community learning disability team. People with learning disabilities are often prescribed medications at different times for various ailments, and as they are often unable to exert their choice by not taking medication, they remain on a varied cocktail. Pharmacists monitor the medications that people are taking and encourage other members of the team to review the need for them. They also advise on the safe storage and administration of medications in residential units. They help to improve compliance by advising on preparations of medications which may be more palatable to the patient, and on ways of administering them without loss of efficacy.

Psychiatrist

A psychiatrist is a qualified medical practitioner who then receives further training in all branches of psychiatry over a 4-year period. After successful completion of the examination to become a Member of the Royal College of Psychiatrists, further training in the psychiatry of learning disability is undertaken for at least 3 years, leading to accreditation as a specialist.

The core roles of the psychiatrist are to provide assessment and treatment for people with a learning disability who have mental illnesses, dementia, behaviour disorders, developmental disorders (e.g. autism) or neuropsychiatric disorders (including epilepsy), and those who come into contact with the courts or the police because of their behaviour. This assessment can be undertaken in a variety of settings, including schools, work settings, people's own homes, outpatient clinics, hospitals and prisons.

Assessment usually leads to a diagnosis of one or more problems and a treatment plan that is drawn up after discussion with other members of the team. Common treatments used by psychiatrists include advice and medication in the management of mental illnesses such as schizophrenia and depression and other conditions such as epilepsy. Psychiatrists are regularly involved in the use of the Mental Health Act to treat some patients who require treatment but are unable to give consent for or refuse it on account of their mental disorder. Other treatments include psychotherapy and advice on behaviour problems. Psychiatrists are also able to advise carers and professionals on issues such as consent to treatment, ability to parent, etc. The service is provided to people of all age groups. The Royal College of Psychiatrists recommends that there should be one consultant psychiatrist for every 100 000 members of the population, although in practice this is rarely the case.

Like other members of the team, the psychiatrist is most effective if working closely with other professionals. Close joint working arrangements often exist for collaboration with psychologists and nurses, with joint assessments and treatments being provided. When this situation exists with behaviour support teams, it becomes possible to diagnose and treat a wide range of mental illnesses that can masquerade as behaviour disorder.

The involvement of the psychiatrist is discussed further in Chapter 14.

Other professionals

Dentists and chiropodists often specialise in working with people with learning disabilities, and provide valuable input to the team. Team members liaise closely with general practitioners, health visitors, paediatricians and district nurses to improve healthcare for people with learning disabilities. Hospital liaison teams will improve the quality of care that learning-disabled people receive in acute hospitals.

Other learning disability teams

In the preceding section an attempt has been made to outline the specific roles of the professionals in the community learning disability team. It is important to emphasise that these professionals also carry out their roles as members of a team in a variety of settings. Multi-disciplinary working is the norm in most patient settings. The latter could be short-term residential assessment and treatment units for adults and children or specialised forensic medium-secure services. In recent years, certain community learning disability teams have specialised further in the client group with which they work, and there are teams for children with a learning disability, and for older adults with a learning disability, as well as community forensic learning disability teams. Some of these are described more fully in Chapter 14.

How do teams work?

The following case study illustrates how teams often approach clinical problems.

Susan is a 31-year-old woman with a moderate learning disability who lives with her family. Her parents are both employed, and during the day she attends a sheltered workshop. The manager of the workshop has referred Susan to the team. According to him Susan has become withdrawn and her level of work has deteriorated. Since her motivation appears to be poor, she is at risk of losing her placement.

At a team meeting the referral is discussed and it is agreed that a community nurse will visit Susan at the day centre and assess the situation. This reveals that Susan has indeed started to deteriorate over the last 3 months. She has Down syndrome and has shown a loss of interest in favourite activities such as cooking, going shopping and meeting her friends. The nurse feels that in order to establish the reason for this change a comprehensive assessment is needed. A full hearing and vision test is performed by the community audiology service and an experienced optician. A referral is made to the general practitioner to examine and investigate Susan for conditions such as anaemia and impaired thyroid functioning. As these tests are found to be negative, a referral is made to the psychologist to measure cognitive functioning in order to rule out early dementia. When this does not reveal any abnormality, Susan is referred for a full psychiatric assessment. This reveals that she is indeed significantly depressed, with loss of weight, loss of appetite, lowered mood and occasional weeping episodes. This was found to have started after her best friend had moved to another centre. This move had not been explained to Susan, and she was under the impression that her friend had died. A short course of antidepressant medication along with resumption of regular contact with her friend leads to a gradual improvement and a return to her previous level of functioning.

This case study demonstrates that multi-disciplinary and multi-agency working is the only way forward to ensure that people with learning disabilities receive appropriate services. No one professional can function independently, and the roles of the different members of the team fit together like the pieces of a jigsaw puzzle.

Acknowledgement

I would like to thank Janet Bailey, Louise Elliot, Liz Kelly, Carlene McKenzie, Sue Marshall, Alan Rudman and Michelle Toorish, who were my colleagues in a community learning disability team, for their help and advice during the preparation of this chapter.

References

Department of Health (2001) *Valuing People: a new strategy for learning disability for the twenty-first century.* Department of Health, London.

McGill P and Toogood S (1994) Organising community placements. In: P McGill and J Mansell (eds) *Severe Learning Disability and Challenging Behaviour: designing high-quality services.* Chapman & Hall, London.

Mansell J (1994) Challenging behaviour: the prospect for change. A keynote review. *Br J Learn Disabil.* **22**: 2–5.

Chapter 14

Towards an integrated health service for people with intellectual disabilities

Ashok Roy and Meera Roy

Understanding health needs

Continuing reforms in the National Health Service have created fundamental changes in the manner in which services are conceptualised, planned and delivered. This chapter describes the different types of services that are available to meet the needs of people with a learning disability who have significant health problems. Lyndsey (2002) has reviewed these services and identified barriers to the provision of appropriate care.

The first set of health problems is encountered in general practice. Common examples include difficulties in seeing and hearing, obesity, hypertension, diabetes and heart disease. There is evidence that people with a learning disability have a higher prevalence of some of these conditions and a lower consultation rate with their general practitioners than the general population (Wilson and Haire 1990; Kerr *et al.* 1996). Lyndsey noted that people with a learning disability and their carers are often unaware of potential health problems, especially if such problems do not cause discomfort or distress. A decline in the level of functioning may be wrongly attributed to the learning disability itself. There are often difficulties in attending the general practitioner's surgery, due to having to wait in a crowded area, and the consultation may be made more difficult due to the communication problems that healthcare professionals encounter when dealing with people with a learning disability. Carers may be dealing with their own feelings about the disabled person, which may have to be dealt with before the client's needs are addressed. Common feelings include guilt, shame and anger. The final result may be that the individual is not thoroughly examined and the condition remains undetected. This combination of factors can lead to health needs not being recognised and met. However, these needs must be taken into account when planning and providing services.

The second set of problems includes a variety of disorders and conditions that are more prevalent in people with a learning disability, and conditions whose manifestation is significantly altered by the presence of a learning disability.

- Psychiatric disorders include the whole range of conditions described in Chapter 3, such as schizophrenia, depression and neurotic disorders (including phobias). These disorders are more frequently encountered in people with a learning disability. They frequently coexist with other physical, developmental and psychosocial factors, and this can make mental disorders more difficult to diagnose and treat. For example, manifestations of depression can change with increasingly severe degrees of learning disability, and episodic screaming and self-injury may indicate a depressed mood. Examples of behaviour disorders include aggression, self-injury, excessive eating and drinking, restlessness and wandering.

- Physical disorders include epilepsy (*see* Chapter 5), cerebral palsy and complex sensory handicaps (*see* Chapter 7). These conditions become more prevalent with increasingly severe degrees of learning disability. Epilepsy is frequently more difficult to diagnose and is often more resistant to treatment. Sensory difficulties have usually been underestimated in people with a learning disability, as they have been difficult to detect and tend to be overlooked. There are several syndromes that are frequently encountered in people with a learning disability with coexisting sensory difficulties. These include Down syndrome, fragile X syndrome and congenital rubella. An individual with Down syndrome may have severe learning disability, congenital heart defects, hearing impairments and dementia.
- Developmental disorders include autism and Asperger's syndrome (*see* Chapter 4).

The third set of health problems is more frequently seen in district general hospitals. Diseases in this broad category are similar to those that affect the general population. Common examples are serious conditions such as chest infections and fractured limbs resulting from injury, which usually need inpatient care. These situations can lead to particular problems for people with a learning disability, because they may not understand what is happening to them and why they have had to leave home and be cared for by unfamiliar people. This could lead to apprehension and lack of cooperation with treatment. Hospital staff are not usually accustomed to dealing with people with a learning disability. They can find it difficult to set aside enough time to communicate effectively and explain what is going on, and they may also find it difficult to explain the reasons for blood tests and other investigations.

Service principles

An influential Government White Paper (Department of Health 2001) highlights the importance of improving access to mainstream services and providing specialist services when mainstream services cannot meet the needs of the population. Local partnership boards, including service planners, providers and users, serve as planning forums for a local area. Guidance has been published on health facilitation and health action plans as a means of improving the health of people with learning disabilities (Department of Health 2002) using the twin approach of accessing family doctors and adopting healthier lifestyles. This new approach – highlighting partnership working – is the underlying principle for a wide range of initiatives summarised in the Government's *Annual Report on Learning Disability* (Department of Health 2004).

Service components

A comprehensive and integrated service would have several key components, each of which will now be considered in turn.

Needs assessment

The first step in planning services is to have an accurate assessment of the needs of the population to be served. It is therefore necessary to identify the population with a learning disability that requires services. This is done by creating a register of service users or by checking the general practitioner lists in the area. Epidemiological data are sometimes used to calculate the figures for a given population.

After the population has been identified, it is essential to know the prevalence of health problems so that the volume and configuration of services can be determined. Estimates can be derived from existing prevalence data. Other methods include surveys from population samples, focus groups or in-depth informant interviews.

Data about coexisting psychiatric, psychological, developmental, physical and psychosocial disabilities in the population can provide an indication of the number of professionals and their skills, the number and range of day services, respite care assessment and treatment facilities and the priorities for service. The size and configuration of the community teams can be determined for a particular catchment area so that they are able to deal with referrals appropriately.

These agencies need to agree priorities for health services and how those services should be provided. Lack of agreement leads to gaps appearing in services and health needs not being met both for individuals and for groups of people. Surveys have shown that only a very small proportion of health authorities provide a full range of services for people with a learning disability (Roy and Cumella 1993).

Prevention

Genetic counselling for families of people with a learning disability aims to reduce the risk of recurrence of the particular condition. The first step in this process is the confirmation of the diagnosis itself. This often involves extensive history taking followed by physical, biochemical, cytogenetic and molecular genetic testing. If the mode of inheritance is known or can be discerned from the family tree, then the risk of recurrence can be determined.

Immunisation against diseases such as rubella which are known to cause severe multiple disabilities has resulted in a marked reduction in the incidence of such births.

Universal screening for disabling conditions such as phenylketonuria is an example of secondary prevention, where the disease is detected at birth and specific interventions such as dietary regimes are put in place to prevent the onset of learning disability. Replacement thyroxine therapy for newborn babies who have been diagnosed with hypothyroidism is an example of a similar strategy.

Examples of prevention aimed at minimising the sequelae of an existing learning disability include regular hearing, visual and thyroid checks in people with Down syndrome, and physiotherapy for children with cerebral palsy. Other strategies, such as access to improved antenatal care, accident prevention and measures to counteract under-stimulating and deprived home environments, should be planned and provided for at-risk groups in the community. Diagnosis and vigorous management of delays in the development of motor and communication skills can help to reduce the adverse physical and psychological effects which may occur.

Improved neonatal care can reduce the onset of disabling conditions, although it can also lead to the increased survival of very-low-birthweight babies, a proportion of whom develop learning disabilities.

Prevention is discussed in more detail in Chapter 2.

Assessment and treatment

Careful assessment is the first step in planning and implementing treatment programmes. This can take place in a variety of settings, such as outpatient clinics, day services, people's own homes or specialised units. Due to the interaction between the individual and the environment it is sometimes important to conduct assessments in different environments.

Assessment

The first step is to obtain a full account of the person's difficulties from their carers. It is essential to obtain information from people who know the individual well. If he or she uses other services, then it would be useful to find out whether the difficulties occur in those settings as well. The information obtained should include early development, schooling, friendships, personality features, current occupation, previous medical history and psychiatric history, including history of any offending behaviour and substance abuse. In addition to a description of the presenting complaints it is important to obtain details of any change in appetite, weight, sleep, excretion, mood and skills.

The degree of disability will influence how an examination may be performed. For more able individuals with good communication skills, this is not significantly different from the procedure for the general population. Such individuals can provide information about the difficulties that led them to seek help. They can also describe their emotions and feelings. As the degree of disability increases, the clinician requires more specialised skills to carry out assessments, and they may need to see the individual on more than one occasion in settings where they may be more at home with someone whom they trust.

The clinician will need to look for evidence suggestive of mental illness. Cognitive disturbance would be manifested by abnormalities in linking thoughts together in a clear sequence and at a normal speed. Disturbances in the content of thinking would be characterised by the presence of delusions, and perceptual abnormalities would include auditory and visual hallucinations. Mood disorders include persistent lowering of mood or mood swings. Passivity phenomena are characterised by feelings of being controlled by external agencies. In the case of individuals with a more severe degree of disability the examiner may have to make deductions from the individual's behaviours. For example, they might undertake a careful examination of patterns of screaming or self-injurious behaviour over a period of time. Behaviour problems can thus be a symptom of a mental illness. They can also serve as a dysfunctional form of communication or the avoidance of a task or situation. Sometimes the behaviour problems are part of a specific syndrome (e.g. Prader–Willi syndrome, Lesch–Nyhan syndrome) (*see* Chapter 6).

The assessment would need to look for evidence of common developmental disorders such as autistic spectrum disorder (ASD) and attention deficit hyper-activity disorder (ADHD) (*see* Chapter 4).

A thorough physical examination is central to any assessments. It should include a measurement of blood pressure and body mass index (BMI), in view of the high prevalence of obesity in people with a learning disability. This should be followed by a comprehensive evaluation of all systems, including the cardiovascular system (heart and blood vessels), respiratory system (lungs), gastrointestinal system (bowel) and central nervous system (brain and spinal cord). Investigations such as full blood count, liver, kidney and thyroid functions and vitamin B_{12} and folate levels should be done routinely. If epileptic activity is suspected, electroencephalograms including ambulatory recordings may be necessary. Brain scans are helpful for determining brain lesions, and this information may help both in localising the causes of disability and in planning treatments.

In order to plan a comprehensive treatment package it is important to have assessments conducted by other members of the multi-disciplinary team (*see* Chapter 13).

Rating scales such as the Hamilton Depression Rating Scale can be used for people with mild learning disabilities. In addition, there are scales such as the Leicester Kettering Scale (Cooper and Collacot 1996) that are specifically designed to detect mood disorders in people with severe learning disabilities. The Psychiatric Assessment Schedules for Adults with Developmental Disabilities (PAS-ADD) were designed to improve the detection and assessment of these disorders in people with intellectual disability (Costello *et al.* 1997; Moss *et al.* 1997). They provide a framework within which clinicians, other healthcare professionals and family members can collect standardised information about symptoms. Checklists are available to assess adaptive and maladaptive behaviour, dementia, ASD and ADHD, and to monitor the efficacy of treatment programmes. They are useful aids to the diagnosis and monitoring of treatments.

As this client group usually has multiple difficulties, the system of multi-axial diagnosis (ICD-10) (World Health Organization 1996) is a useful way of listing the areas of concern. This system consists of the following axes:

- Axis I – severity of learning disability and problem behaviours
- Axis II – associated medical conditions
- Axis III – associated psychiatric and developmental disorders
- Axis IV – global assessment of psychosocial disability
- Axis V – associated abnormal psychosocial situations.

This system ensures that all of the difficulties are dealt with appropriately by basing treatment plans on the needs highlighted by the multi-axial diagnosis.

Treatment

A comprehensive diagnosis ensures that all of the problems are dealt with systematically. People with learning disabilities often have undiagnosed hearing and visual problems. Correction in these areas will obviously improve their quality of life. Obesity and vitamin deficiencies should be corrected both by providing supplements and in the long term by giving advice on healthy eating. Thyroid dysfunction is common in people with Down syndrome. Impaired hepatic and renal function may have a bearing on long-term treatment with anticonvulsants and lithium.

People with learning disabilities and additional mental illness respond to the pharmacological therapies that are available to the general population. They require drugs in the usual therapeutic range if these are to be of benefit. Carbamazepine and sodium valproate are often used to stabilise recurrent mood disorders, and an advantage of these drugs over lithium is that it is easier to maintain therapeutic levels without relying on blood tests, as some people with learning disabilities are extremely distressed by blood tests. As in the general population, depot preparations of antipsychotic drugs have an advantage over oral preparations in that they improve compliance. The use of stimulant drugs such as methylphenidate for people of all ages diagnosed with ADHD has yielded encouraging results.

A significant number of people with learning disabilities have seizure disorders, and improved control of epilepsy is an important part of treatment. The underlying brain damage means that control of epilepsy often requires more than one anticonvulsant. Even with the use of long-acting preparations and the newer anticonvulsants it is sometimes impossible to eliminate seizures altogether. Some anticonvulsants can cause impairments in cognitive functioning.

The treatment of physical disorders must be an integral part of the comprehensive care package. Usually this requires interventions by other medical and surgical specialists. As psychiatric and physical difficulties are only part of the learning-disabled person's problem, multi-disciplinary care packages are the cornerstone of treatment programmes. For example, eating problems are common in this client group, and interventions by dietitians can be extremely helpful. As the affected person may have physical disabilities, an occupational therapist may be able to advise on suitable utensils, drinking cups, etc. Together with physiotherapists, they can improve seating and mobility. They can also advise carers on aids and appliances that can be used at home, safe lifting and handling techniques, and increased independence. Physiotherapists are able to improve and maintain mobility by means of hydrotherapy, etc. As communication difficulties often contribute to behaviour difficulties, any aids to improving communication should improve behaviours, and therefore communication therapists make important contributions to care packages (*see* Chapter 13 for a more detailed account of multi-disciplinary working).

Behaviour difficulties may be the result of environmental difficulties. It may be that the individual is not at ease with particular fellow residents, in which case a move away from the person concerned may improve behaviour. People with autism are happier in a structured and predictable environment with a high staff:client ratio. Thus a close examination of environmental issues and their manipulation will pay dividends in improving behaviours.

Family interactions are also important, as certain behavioural difficulties may occur only at home and not at the day centre or school. This may be due to the carers being inconsistent in their approach to the individual, and some advice on this could improve the situation. As there are often unresolved grief issues, family therapy can be beneficial. Interventions to reduce expressed emotions will improve the outcome for individuals with additional mental health problems.

Cognitive and behavioural approaches are useful, as are relaxation techniques, anxiety management, anger management and structured behaviour programmes. Learning-disabled people may also benefit from individual counselling and group work that addresses personal relationships and sexuality issues. More specialised groups for fire setters and sexual offenders are held in forensic learning disability units.

Following the Community Care Act 1991, care management has become widely used in learning disability services. The care manager undertakes a comprehensive assessment of the person's needs, including health needs, and draws up a care package involving the individual, their carers and relevant professionals. The care manager then commissions the care from statutory or independent-sector providers using funding from social services and/or primary care trusts, depending on whether the needs are due to social factors, health factors, or a combination of both.

The care programme approach (CPA) is a useful Government initiative for delivering mental health services, and it has been adopted by specialist learning disability services. For people with a straightforward mental health need, a basic CPA may suffice. More commonly the person's needs are complex and an enhanced CPA is required. The CPA assessment is similar to the assessment under care management, and results in a care coordinator being appointed. As people with learning disabilities are also liable to receive treatments under the Mental Health Act 1983, the CPA assessment may suggest a supervised discharge or a guardianship (Roy 2000) for a detained patient.

The assessment and treatment of people with learning disabilities and additional health needs are eclectic and draw on the methods used in other branches of psychiatry and medicine. As health problems are only part of the whole picture, both the assessment and the care package must be multi-disciplinary (*see* Chapter 13).

Improved care from general practitioners

There are several methods of improving the quality of care that general practitioners provide for people with a learning disability and their carers. Studies have shown that many GPs do not have adequate information about services for people with a learning disability in their local area (Marshall *et al.* 1996). Closure of hospital services and the development of community-based facilities have led to local service provision being in a state of transition. General practitioners must be updated regularly on the local facilities and community teams. Sometimes they may not have much information about the people with a learning disability on their list and their current health status. It has been shown that comprehensive and regular health checks lead to the detection of a range of health problems, such as obesity, hypertension, diabetes, ear problems, drug toxicity, dental caries and hypothyroidism (Martin *et al.* 1997). Most of the conditions detected are easily treated at the GP's surgery, but sometimes referral to specialist services is necessary. Attention is drawn to the health of the carers and their ability to cope. Support can be sought from respite care schemes and the local community teams. Strong working links between the GPs and their staff on the one hand and the community learning disability teams on the other can provide an umbrella of services to meet the health needs of people with a learning disability. Health facilitation (Department of Health 2002) has proved to be a useful vehicle for coordinating these initiatives.

Mental health services

In order to meet the mental health needs of people with learning disabilities, services must be comprehensive and flexible. The most important professional group that provides a service is the learning disability team (*see* Chapter 13). Psychiatrists, psychologists, nurses and other therapists can jointly assess and meet the majority of the mental health needs of people with a learning disability. Assessments and treatment are often likely to occur in the individual's home or workplace. The aim of assessment is to reach an accurate diagnosis and a better understanding of the individual's problems. This then helps the team to work with the individual to produce a treatment plan that addresses all of the main problems. Effective interventions can lead to improvements which can be measured using outcome scales such as the Health of the Nation Outcome Scales for People with Learning Disabilities (Roy *et al.* 2002). The duration of treatment is variable, and in some instances can take several months or even years. For example, the treatment of an uncomplicated depressive illness or a temporary loss of seizure control in an individual with epilepsy may be completed within a few weeks. In contrast, the implementation of a management strategy for an individual with a severe learning disability, autism and severe self-injurious behaviour may take years to produce measurable change.

In general, professionals working in learning disability services provide psychiatric services for people with a severe learning disability. For people with a mild learning disability it is possible to provide a service jointly with staff from general psychiatry services. Team members working jointly can share knowledge and facilities to meet the needs of this client group. However, in people with a significant level of learning disability the staff in mainstream mental health services may not have the expertise necessary to deal with the complex mental disorders that are frequently encountered. Integrated models of working have been developed in which a range of responses from both services lead to a successful outcome.

Sometimes it is necessary to move the individual from his or her normal environment to a specialised unit for more comprehensive interventions. The various settings are considered below.

Home and work

In this situation, the person with a mental health need is assessed in familiar surroundings in order to look for factors that precipitate, exacerbate and maintain problem behaviours. For example, nurses, psychologists and behaviour therapists can make observations and make environmental changes in a systematic way in an attempt to modify behaviour. They can also educate carers about mental disorders and improve their understanding of the problems.

Outpatient clinics

Psychiatrists commonly work in this setting. History taking, mental and physical examinations and investigations can be undertaken here. Treatments such as advice, counselling and psychotherapy are also provided. Joint working between psychiatrists and other professionals is usual, as are joint clinics with other specialists such as paediatricians, neurologists and geneticists.

Day services

Intensive, multi-professional assessments and treatments are sometimes undertaken in specialised, well-staffed day units which provide opportunities for assessment, treatment, training and education. This allows an opportunity to monitor the effects of treatment, working with carers and families, and provides support with regard to accessing community facilities as well as leisure and work.

Inpatient units

When psychiatric and behavioural problems are too severe or dangerous to manage at home, it may be necessary to move the individual to specialised residential assessment and treatment facilities for varying periods of time. Sometimes this may be done on an involuntary basis by using the Mental Health Act when the individual is a danger to him- or herself or others on account of a mental disorder (the Act is discussed in Chapter 11). Common reasons for admission would be behaviour problems such as severe aggression or self-injury, severe mental illnesses, offending behaviour and severe epilepsy requiring urgent medication review. Specialised well-trained multi-disciplinary teams are able to offer 24-hour assessment and treatment of the individual by providing close observation and supervision, initiating new types of treatment and, in some cases, providing a secure and predictable environment. It would be possible, for instance, to commence treatment with a different drug (e.g. lithium or clozapine) which needs very close monitoring initially. It can also help to examine emotional relationships within families and provide an opportunity for planning the future.

Inpatient treatment could occur in a specialist learning disability psychiatry unit, a generic adult psychiatry unit, a unit with shared staffing, smaller community base units, single patient units or in mental nursing homes. The key to success is an effective well-supported team that can work in partnership with clients and their families.

An important part of coordinating and providing a comprehensive service to a population with diverse and complicated health needs is joint working with professionals in other services. These include other psychiatric specialties such as child psychiatry and forensic psychiatry, and other medical personnel such as paediatricians, school doctors and dentists. Good joint working can lead to the development of *specialised services*, which are described below.

Services for children and adolescents with mental health needs

The starting point for this service is clear agreements and joint working between psychiatrists in learning disability and the community learning disability teams, child psychiatrists, paediatricians and the children's services. The health services then need to work closely with social services and education. Community paediatricians working with specialised teams in child developmental centres usually detect children with generalised developmental delay. There should be good links between these centres and local disability teams. If the learning disability is apparent at birth (e.g. Down's syndrome), the learning disability teams can provide advice and support to the family at an early stage. If the disability is not apparent in early life or there is parental reluctance to accept the disability, there may be a delay in the involvement of the learning disability teams. Early intervention can be of help with sleep problems, incontinence, overactivity and self-injury. Children with significant emotional and behaviour problems need help from psychiatrists and psychologists from both services, together with education service staff, nurses and social workers. There needs to be clarity among teachers and parents about how to access appropriate services. Clarity is also needed between mental health services and child health services with regard to the management of children with coexisting physical disorders such as epilepsy, cerebral palsy and congenital heart disease.

Adolescents with learning disability and mental health problems often find it difficult to access appropriate services due to poor coordination between learning disability, general psychiatry and forensic psychiatry services and sometimes services for people with autism.

Services for people with ASD and ADHD

As was mentioned in Chapter 4, people with autism and other pervasive developmental disorders can develop emotional and behaviour problems. Depression, anxiety, aggression, self-injury and psychotic disorders have recently been reported in this population. In order to deal with these problems, the whole range of assessment and treatment services must be made available. There are some specific issues that need to be borne in mind. The main features of autism (impaired communication skills, poor social interactions and restricted stereo-typical behaviour) can themselves mimic various mental illnesses, such as obsessive-compulsive disorder, depression and psychotic conditions. The communication problem often makes it difficult to elicit the symptoms of illness. Another problem is that a varying degree of learning disability often coexists, which must be assessed and taken into account when planning treatment. Treatments are more difficult to implement, as drugs sometimes have idiosyncratic and paradoxical effects. For example, tranquillisers may cause excitement and restlessness. Behavioural treatments can be difficult to generalise, so that strategies which work in one setting (e.g. the clinic) do not work in another (e.g. at home). This can make progress with treatment slow and more labour-intensive. Consistency of the environment and in handling, together with a predictable routine, is essential if progress is to be made with assessment and treatment. A further problem is that because of the poor social skills, effective treatment cannot be provided easily in group settings, and most long-term treatment programmes must be individually tailored. In some instances of severe psychiatric and behavioural problems, change is very slow and strategies must be devised to reduce the risks to the individual and those around them while maximising opportunities to develop and have a good quality of life. It is vital that staff working in these services have a good understanding of autism and mental illnesses so that they can understand the individuals for whom they are caring and thus make effective care plans.

Undiagnosed ADHD is associated with behaviour problems which can be refractory to conventional treatment and may need the administration of psychostimulants for successful management.

Case study

A 16-year-old boy was referred for inpatient assessment and treatment from a special school for autistic children for the management of epilepsy and severe self-injurious behaviour. His anti-epileptic medication was reviewed and his seizures were reduced. After careful observation over a period of 3 months it became apparent that some of his self-injurious behaviour was a symptom of an underlying mood disorder (depression), as it increased when he looked sad, lost his appetite and had sleep disturbance. Other self-injurious behaviours were only present when he was asked to engage in activities which he did not feel like doing at the time. Treatment with lithium resulted in a reduction of the periodic self-injury. Exploration of his likes and dislikes and improved planning of his day services with a reduction in the amount of group activities led to a reduction in the self-injurious behaviour, which had a task avoidance role.

Services for people with personality abnormalities

This is a heterogeneous group of people who have deeply ingrained and enduring behaviour patterns that affect multiple domains of their lives, such as psychological, social, occupational and interpersonal functioning. Common types of personality abnormality that are encountered in services include people with emotionally unstable and dissocial personality disorders. Assessment and treatment are difficult and time consuming because the diagnosis is not widely used. There appears to be diagnostic overshadowing from mental illnesses which may also coexist. The differentiation is important because although antipsychotic medications are useful in the treatment of various mental illnesses, they are of more limited benefit in the management of personality disorders, and are usually used as adjuncts to psychological and behavioural treatments.

Lithium, carbamazepine and sodium valproate are useful in the management of mood swings and aggression. Anti-psychotic drugs have been used for the reduction of anger. Antidepressants have been used in the management of associated depression, and anti-libidinal drugs are used as part of the treatment of sex offenders. Anti-anxiety drugs have been used for short periods to control anxiety.

Psychological measures that are commonly used include social skills training, anger management and psychotherapeutic approaches (e.g. cognitive therapy). These treatments are usually provided along with opportunities for education and work.

Services for offenders

Services for people with a learning disability who exhibit offending behaviour need to take into account the level of learning disability, the nature of the offence and the degree of security required. People with mild learning disability can receive their treatment from general forensic services. However, if the learning disability is significant, the individual will need input from forensic learning disability specialists. The relationship between offending behaviour, mental illness and behaviour disorders can be represented diagrammatically as shown in Figure 14.1.

There are significant overlaps that must be borne in mind when assessing and treating people who exhibit offending behaviour. A comprehensive assessment focuses on psychiatric status, personality traits, educational attainment, social skills, relationships, employment and leisure opportunities. An individual with a depressive illness and communication difficulty may display aggression, which in turn may be manifested as offending behaviour such as fire setting. Failure to diagnose and treat the depression is likely to lead to recurrent offending. It is not

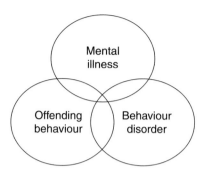

Figure 14.1 Links between mental illness, offending behaviour and behaviour disorder.

uncommon for a person with an emotionally unstable personality disorder to be involved in assaults against others. This behaviour may improve in response to relaxation and anger management as well as engaging in structured supported daytime occupation.

Specific treatment programmes have been designed to help people with a learning disability who have committed arson and sexual offences. The treatment programmes are based on those provided for people without a learning disability, and have been modified for use in this population. The treatment is given to carefully screened and selected groups. It aims to help the individual to acknowledge his or her problem, understand the reasons for offending, devise strategies and use them to reduce the rate of re-offending.

Community teams, specialised forensic teams, the probation service and social services deal with people with a learning disability who commit offences. These individuals can often be diverted from courts to the health service by close coordination between the police, the courts and healthcare professionals. In many instances the assessment and treatment can be carried out in the community. In the case of more serious offences, increasing levels of supervision will be necessary. Facilities that provide more security, such as regional secure units and special hospitals, are described in Chapter 12. An individual's dangerousness must be continually assessed, and the level of security required needs to be matched to the risk that the individual poses. After treatment, individuals can move from secure facilities with perimeter fencing to less secure, well-staffed units, eventually moving to the community with support.

Services for elderly people with a learning disability

As people with a learning disability grow older, they find it hard to access mainstream services for the elderly due to their intellectual and communication difficulties. People with Down syndrome tend to age prematurely, and need to be under regular surveillance to ensure that problems such as hearing and visual defects, thyroid disorders and dementia are detected early. Some of these issues are discussed further in Chapter 11.

General hospital services

Staff in general hospitals need to receive training to increase their awareness of the nature of the health and communication difficulties that people with learning disabilities may experience. There needs to be more awareness of the difficulties involved in obtaining informed consent. This means that the planned treatment must be explained in a manner appropriate to the person's communication ability. Verbal communication may have to be supported by the use of signs and symbols. Some treatments may be more difficult to explain than others. For example, a dental extraction may be easier to explain than a complex treatment involving a combination of drugs for a chronic bowel disease. It must also be remembered that if an adult with a learning disability is unable to give informed consent, no other individual can give consent on his or her behalf. In these circumstances the treatment will then need to be discussed with individuals who are involved with the learning-disabled person and carried out in that person's best interests. The situation is more complex if the treatment will affect the person's ability to have children (*see* Chapter 13).

Agreements should be in place with local hospitals for access to beds for both planned and emergency treatments. Community learning disability teams can provide support for people with a learning disability who are using outpatient and inpatient facilities. Support is also needed to access X-ray departments and laboratories for investigations.

Priorities for the future

One of the most important issues to be resolved in service planning and delivery in the future is that of coordination between health services and social services. Social services are regarded as the lead agency for services for people with a learning disability. In dealing with people with additional health needs, there is a need for clarity of roles and responsibilities between the agencies. Lack of clarity has led to delay in the provision of services and patchy service development with inevitable wasting of resources. A shared understanding of health needs, responsibility in planning and provision and the pooling of resources may aid the development of comprehensive, responsive and local services.

A second priority area is the need to increase the involvement of general practitioners in the delivery of services. This involves further raising of awareness of the health needs of this population, along with more information about the specialised services that are available and closer working between them and community learning disability teams.

A third priority is to make families and carers as well as all staff working in learning disability services (e.g. schools and day centres) aware of the health needs of people with a learning disability. Lack of knowledge of health problems can lead to serious consequences such as worsening of health, and erroneous attribution of this to the learning disability itself. Behaviour problems and other changes in health status must trigger a full assessment and appropriate treatment.

The publication of the document *Signposts for Success in Commissioning and Providing Health Services for People with Learning Disabilities* (Department of Health 1998) has provided comprehensive guidelines for good practice in shaping health services for the future.

References

Cooper SA and Collacot RA (1996) Depressive episodes in adults with learning disability. *Ir J Psychol Med.* **13:** 105–13.

Costello H, Moss SC, Prosser H and Hatton C (1997) Reliability of the ICD-10 version of the Psychiatric Assessment Schedule for Adults with Developmental Disability (PAS-ADD). *Soc Psychiatry Psychiatr Epidemiol.* **32**: 339–43.

Department of Health (1998) *Signposts for Success in Commissioning and Providing Health Services for People with Learning Disabilities.* Department of Health, London.

Department of Health (2001) *Valuing People: a new strategy for learning disability for the twenty-first century.* Department of Health, London.

Department of Health (2002) *Action for Health, Health Action Plans and Health Facilitation: detailed good practice guidance on implementation for learning disability partnership boards.* Department of Health, London.

Department of Health (2004) *Valuing People: moving forward together. The Government Annual Report on Learning Disability.* Department of Health, London.

Kerr MP, Richards D and Glover G (1996) Primary care for people with an intellectual disability: a group practice survey. *J Appl Res Intellect Disabil.* **9**: 347–52.

Lyndsey MP (2002) Comprehensive health care services for people with learning disabilities. *Adv Psychiatr Treat.* **8**: 138–47.

Marshall S, Martin DM and Myles F (1996) Survey of GPs' views of learning disability services. *Br J Nurs.* **5**: 488–93.

Martin DM, Roy A and Wells MB (1997) Health gains through health checks: improving access to primary health care for people with intellectual disability. *J Intellect Disabil Res.* **41**: 401–8.

Moss SC, Ibbotson B, Prosser H, Goldberg DP, Patel P and Simpson N (1997) Validity of the PAS-ADD for detecting psychiatric symptoms in adults with learning disability. *Soc Psychiatry Psychiatr Epidemiol.* **32**: 344–54

Roy A (2000) The Care Programme Approach in learning disability psychiatry. *Adv Psychiatr Treat.* **6**: 380–87.

Roy A, Clifford P, Mathews H, Martin DM and Fowler V (2002) Health of the Nation Outcome Scales for People with Learning Disabilities (HoNOS-LD). Glossary for HoNOS-LD score sheet. *Br J Psychiatry.* **180**: 67–70.

Roy A and Cumella S (1993) Developing local services for people with a learning disability and a psychiatric disorder. *Psychiatr Bull.* **17**: 215–17.

Wilson DN and Haire A (1990) Health care screening for people with mental handicap living in the community. *BMJ.* **301**: 1379–81.

World Health Organization (1996) *ICD-10 Guide for Mental Retardation.* World Health Organization, Geneva.

Further reading

Department of Health (1992) *Health Services for People with Learning Disabilities (Mental Handicap).* Department of Health, London.

Department of Health (1992) *Social Care for Adults with Learning Disabilities (Mental Handicap).* Department of Health, London.

Department of Health (1995) *The Health of the Nation: a strategy for people with learning disabilities.* HMSO, London.

Department of Health (1998) *Signposts for Success in Commissioning and Providing Health Services for People with Learning Disabilities.* Department of Health, London.

Royal College of Psychiatrists (1997) *Meeting the Mental Health Needs of People with Learning Disabilities. Part I. Adults with mild learning disability. Part II. Elderly people with learning disabilities.* Royal College of Psychiatrists, London.

Index

Page numbers in italics refer to figures or tables.